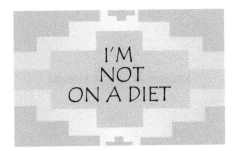

I'M
NOT
ON A DIET

I'M NOT ON A DIET

Culture, Health and Healing

Natalia Medina Coggins
and
Kip Coggins

SUNSTONE
PRESS

Santa Fe

Sunstone books may be purchased for educational, business, or sales promotional use. For information please write: Special Markets Department, Sunstone Press, P.O. Box 2321, Santa Fe, New Mexico 87504-2321.

Book and Cover design ◉ Vicki Ahl
Body typeface ◉ Palatino Linotype
Printed on acid free paper

Library of Congress Cataloging-in-Publication Data

Coggins, Natalia Medina, 1957-
    I'm not on a diet : culture, health and healing / by Natalia Medina Coggins and Kip Coggins.
        p. cm.
    Includes bibliographical references.
    ISBN 978-0-86534-767-0 (softcover : alk. paper)
    1. Nutrition. 2. Food habits. 3. Mexican Americans--Food. 4. Indians of North America--Food. 5. Health. I. Coggins, Kip, 1956- II. Title.
    RA784.C5655 2010
    613.2--dc22

                                    2010013360

Published in

WWW.SUNSTONEPRESS.COM
SUNSTONE PRESS / POST OFFICE BOX 2321 / SANTA FE, NM 87504-2321 /USA
(505) 988-4418 / ORDERS ONLY (800) 243-5644 / FAX (505) 988-1025

This book is dedicated to my mother, Carmen A. Medina. Because of her 20-year battle with Type-2 Diabetes, I was determined to find the nutritional balance in my life.

CONTENTS

About The Authors

Natalia Medina Coggins was born and raised in Chicago, Illinois. Natalia made Albuquerque, New Mexico her home in the spring of 2008. She first moved to the southwest, in August 1993, when her parents retired to El Paso, Texas. After completing her bachelor's degree in psychology, and graduating with honors from the University of Texas at El Paso in December 2000, she has worked exclusively as an editor of articles and texts focusing in the field of social work. Her commitment to helping her mother, who was a Type 2 Diabetic, in understanding the relationships between food and health and becoming health literate was an important step in understanding this "lifestyle" disease. In the fall 1999, after facing health-related issues of her own, Natalia's research into culture and tradition in relation to food became instrumental in the completion of this book and guided her in understanding the natural relationship between culture, health, and healing. She has one daughter, Jessica, who currently lives in the Chicago area.

Kip Coggins was born and raised in northern Michigan and made the southwest his permanent home in the late 1980s, where he has worked, as a social worker, in the Albuquerque and Santa Fe areas. In the fall 1995, he moved to El Paso, Texas where he worked at the University of

Texas at El Paso (UTEP), Social Work Program as a lecturer. After completing his dual doctorate degree in social work and cultural anthropology from the University of Michigan in December 1996, Kip became an assistant professor with the UTEP, Social Work Program. In the fall 2001, Kip was tenured and promoted to associate professor, and served as the program director until the fall 2006. He continues to teach social work at the university level in New Mexico. He has a strong commitment to examining the connection between diet and health among peoples of the southwest. He continues to work with communities within the El Paso, Texas and northern New Mexico areas.

Introduction

Our Growing Health Crisis

Growing Trends in Health-Related Diseases

Currently in the United States, we are experiencing a growing health crisis. Unfortunately, the growing health crisis, is not limited to our country, but is spreading worldwide. Many countries around the world face serious issues related to the health of their citizens, as well. With the dramatic rise in health-related diseases, such as cancer, cardiovascular heart disease, obesity, and diabetes, the United States and many other countries will face economic hardships in trying to provide adequate healthcare. Although, innovations in medical technology do help some; many are not able to access healthcare in their communities, many simply cannot afford the healthcare they need to prevent the devastating effects of many chronic diseases, while others do not have any healthcare insurance to help cover the preventative costs of disease. In looking at current health trends in national and international studies, we will look at why many of these chronic diseases need to be addressed and why policies need to be in place to provide preventative measures to combat the growing epidemic.

According to two independent studies released in 2008, by Duke University researchers and the International Agency for

Research on Cancer (IARC) reported the dramatic rise in both Type 2 Diabetes and Cancer rates will create a worldwide crisis. Both studies showed that if the trends continue, not only will the United States (U.S.) health care systems, but the world health care systems will face an enormous burden in providing medical care. The security and viability of health care systems worldwide are at risk because of the growing number of people affected with these two diseases and their complications. The American Cancer Society (ACS) 2008 Annual Report, the ACS is also concerned with the growing number of new cancer cases, especially for those 25 million in the U.S. who are underinsured, those 47 million in the U.S. with no health insurance, and those who belong to underserved populations, such as Native Americans. Also, in the American Heart Association (AHA) 2009 report, entitled "Heart Disease and Stroke Statistics—2009 Update," show that progress has been made in controlling several of the risk factors, such as high blood pressure and high cholesterol, which are associated with heart disease and stroke. Despite the promising decline in the number of deaths, this trend is in danger of being reversed because of the lack of progress made with other risk factors, such as obesity, diabetes, and lack of physical activity.

The study released in early 2008, by Duke University researchers, dealt with the rise of diabetes and the complications associated with this disease among the elderly in the United States. This study looked at all Medicare cases of diabetes among those over the age of 65 from 1994–1995 to 2003–2004. Within this age group, it was found that new cases rose by 23%, while the prevalence of the disease rose by 62% during the same period. In looking further into the data, researchers found that those diagnosed with diabetes, also had related complications, such as heart disease and stroke. Of those diagnosed with diabetes, 90% had at least one diabetes-related complication within six years after the initial diagnosis. Also, approximately half of those still living at the end of the study had a secondary diagnosis of congestive heart failure. Surprisingly, after being diagnosed with diabetes, the death rate for those diagnosed as a diabetic were 8.3% higher than those not diagnosed and treated for the disease.

In their 2008 Annual Report, the ACS found that although the number of cancer cases and cancer deaths decreased for the first time in a decade, several types of cancer actually increased during the same period. The decline in new cancer cases and cancer deaths are found in three of the most common types of cancers in men: lung cancer, colon cancer, and prostate cancer, and in two of the most common cancers found in women: breast cancer and colon cancer, while there was a leveling off of lung cancer death rates for women. While this is good news, there were several types of cancer which had an increase in new cases, which include cancer of the skin, kidney cancer, and thyroid cancer. Although lung cancer in smokers has shown a dramatic decrease, cigarette smokers account for approximately one third of all cancer deaths in the U.S. While lung cancer deaths have actually decreased in men, lung cancer deaths have increased in 13 states among women.

The growing number of new cancer cases is of concern to the ACS, along with the number of those uninsured, underinsured, and those populations underserved. The ACS believes that there are other interrelated issues that create a lack of access to early diagnosis and treatment of cancer. Many of the newer cancer screening tests are not covered adequately or are not covered at all by insurance companies and therefore must be paid out-of-pocket by those requesting the tests. With the rising costs of medical treatments, many of these existing tests are underused. They cite colon cancer as an example of this type of preventative measure. Colon cancer can be detected when approximately 90% of the cases are curable, while only half of those adults 50 years and older get the colon cancer screening done when recommended. Also, the medical system tends to focus on cancer treatment, once the disease is diagnosed, and the amount of monies made available for cancer research is not adequately funded. However, the ACS believes that the focus needs to be placed on the education and prevention of cancer, with more emphasis on eating a healthy diet, maintaining a healthy body weight, and getting more physical activity.

In the study released in late 2008, the International Agency for Research on Cancer (IARC) looked into the potential global crisis because of the growing incidence of cancer diagnosis. It was reported that cancer is on its way in the leading cause of death by 2010. One of the findings in this report project that new cancer diagnoses will continue to increase by 1% every year. Another finding showed that smoking and lifestyle factors, such as obesity, will overtake chronic infection as the leading cause of cancer, especially in those populations that are poor and from middle-income countries. It is estimated that approximately 1.3 billion people smoke tobacco worldwide and 12% of cancer cases in low-income countries are attributed to the use of tobacco. Not surprisingly, this figure is expected to rise. In looking at some data from different countries, it was found that in India chewing tobacco is an important cancer risk factor. In Japan, Singapore, and Korea breast cancer rates have doubled or tripled over the last four decades. The IARC report stated that worldwide, by the year 2030 there will be 27 million new cancer cases and 17 million cancer-related deaths each year. Worldwide the rate of cancer cases has doubled between 1975 and 2000, and is expected to doubled again by 2020 and triple by 2030.

Costs in Health-Related Diseases

Every ten years, the Department of Health and Human Services (HHS) produces a report which is much like a prospective census which sets goals in 28 health related areas. Some of the specific areas include weight and diabetes incidence, cholesterol levels, and cancer screenings. This report also tracks how well we are meeting the goals set within the ten year period. The next "Healthy People" report is due in 2010, but the HHS released an interim assessment in 2008. According to this assessment, while 59% of its health objectives have been met or on their way to being met, 20% of their health objectives have retreated from the objectives that were set. Some of these statistics are troubling. For example, this assessment reports that in 2003-2006 only 33% of Americans were at a healthy weight; half the number who should be at their ideal weight and 10% fewer than in 1997. In looking at specific diseases, health officials had hoped to cap the prevalence of diabetes at 25 cases per 1,000 people. But currently this number has more than doubled this goal and has actually risen since 1997.

The United States spends far more on health care than any other developed nation. In the U.S., the total annual healthcare spending per capita is $7,026 and is expected to rise because of the increasing number of chronic diseases. In comparison, for example both France and Canada provides government run healthcare for all its citizens. Both of these countries have a lower annual healthcare spending per capita, at $4,056 and $3,912 respectively, than the U.S. While many may argue that the majority of this expense keeps the U.S. a leader in medical innovation, the U.S. still does not have equality of healthcare for all of its citizens.

The cost of U.S. health care is expected to be one-fifth of our national economy within nine years; is expected to double per person and approximately half the money needed for healthcare in the U.S. is expected to come from public assistance programs, like Medicare. For example, hospital care remains the largest expense, especially among the aging population. For every dollar the U.S. spends, $0.31 goes toward hospital care, $0.21 to physician and clinical care, $0.10 to prescription drugs, $0.09 to nursing home care, which includes home healthcare workers, and $0.07 to administrative costs. The remaining costs go toward dental care and medical equipment both at $0.04, research at $0.02, and all other healthcare costs not listed at $0.12. In the coming years, with the large number of baby boomers set to retire, this issue will become more relevant.

The Commonwealth Fund, a foundation which funds healthcare research, reported in 2005 that Americans paid 16% of our gross domestic product (GDP) for healthcare, for a total of $2 trillion. This makes the U.S. the top spender on healthcare per capita in the world. In comparison, France paid 11.1% of its GDP and Canada paid 10% of its GDP. Although the U.S. spends a record amount of money on healthcare, we do not spend it wisely and with equality to all Americans. According to the Commonwealth Fund 2008 report, 101,000 deaths from 2002-2003 could have been avoided with access to timely and effective healthcare. These deaths were from a variety of illnesses that are deemed preventable, such as influenza, pneumonia, diabetes, and stroke. This foundation also reported that in 2005 half of Americans did not receive recommended preventative healthcare, such as vaccinations, cancer screenings, and routine examinations. It was noted that one of the reasons we rank poorly among industrialized nations in delivering healthcare is because we do not have or provide basic wellness infrastructure. Healthcare providers do not focus on preventative measures, but rather focus on treatment of conditions and diseases after the condition has progressed to a more advanced stage. Although not all of these deaths would have been prevented, many health conditions are preventable. While others can be fixed or treated with more success before they become life threatening. As an industrialized nation, we rank last (19th) in providing quality healthcare to our citizens.

The American Diabetes Association (ADA), in an annual report looked at both the direct and indirect costs of diabetes. Type 2 Diabetes is one of the most disabling of diseases because many people are not aware that they are diabetic until they show symptoms of one of the complications. Type 2 Diabetes can lead to numerous complications, which include heart disease and stroke, eye complications which can lead to blindness, kidney disease and kidney failure, nervous system disease which includes complications related to poor circulation, such as amputations, dental disease with the most common periodontal or gum disease, complications of pregnancy, and sexual dysfunction. Controlling diabetes can reduce the risks of developing complications. According to the Department of Health and Human Services (DHHS), adult onset diabetes has a strong physiological tie to cardiovascular heart (CVD). The DHHS also reported that the majority of those diagnosed with Type 2 Diabetes, die from complications of CVD and not from causes directly associated with blood glucose control.

According to the ADA, the annual per capita costs of treating a person with diabetes is $11,744 and one of every five healthcare dollars is spent on caring for a person with diabetes. In 2007 the Center for Disease Control (CDC) reported 8% of Americans or 23.6 million are diabetic, of which 17.9 million are diagnosed diabetics and 5.7 million are undiagnosed. A staggering 57 million are pre-diabetic and likely to become diabetic unless they make life changes. In 2007, 1.6 million new cases were diagnosed for adults 20 years and older. With the numbers increasing, the amount we spend on the treatment of diabetes will continue to rise, as well.

Also, in 2007 the ADA report indicated the total annual economic cost for diabetes in the U.S. was approximately $174 billion. In their report, it stated that medical expenditures totaled $116 billion, of which $27 billion for direct diabetes care, $58 billion for treatment of diabetes-related chronic complications, and $31 billion for excess general medical costs. The remaining $58 billion was spent on indirect costs, of which $26.9 billion represents the value of lost productivity because of premature death-related diabetes. The indirect costs represent other issues, such as diabetes-related unemployment disability, reduced work performance, lost productivity because of early mortality, and increased absenteeism. Unfortunately, the actual cost of this disease cannot be fully calculated because this does not measure pain and suffering, care provided by non-paid caregivers (who are usually family members that must quit their paying jobs to care for a loved one), and the cost of extreme and excessive medical treatment in conjunction with undiagnosed diabetes.

Causes of "Lifestyle" Diseases

Many researchers and health professionals disagree as to some of the direct causes, such as diet, exercise, family history. For example, some researchers believe we may have "genes" that can cause a higher chance to develop certain diseases despite precautions one takes. Recently, researchers from the University of Texas, Southwestern Medical Center found what they believe to be a gene that is linked to serious liver disease, which may lead to the development of other liver diseases, such as cirrhosis and liver failure. This disease, known as Nonalcoholic Fatty Liver Disease (NAFLD), is the most common liver disease in the United States and Europe. Approximately a third of all Americans have fatty livers, a predisposition linked to their ancestry, and may develop NAFLD. Researchers discovered a gene related to liver fat, but with unknown function, called PNPLA3. One variant of this gene does not allow it to function or to function poorly. This gene variant is found in approximately 49% of Hispanics, 23% of European-Americans, and only 17% of African-Americans in the study. While another variant of this same gene links it to lower risk of liver fat. This healthier gene variant was found more often in African-Americans, than in Americans of any other ancestry in the study. Although this research does not conclusively prove that those with fatty liver will develop more serious liver diseases, this gene variant does show an increased susceptibility of diseases of the liver and liver injury.

Another example of a gene that may cause obesity and diabetes is with the Pima Indians in southern Arizona. According to National Institute for Health (NIH), they were initially using the "thrifty gene" theory to help explain why Pima Indians were overweight. This gene was supposed to help the body store fat and then use it in times of famine. Unfortunately, as the Pima Indians adopted a Western lifestyle, which included less physical activity and a diet higher in fat, and with greater access to high calorie foods, this gene started to work against them. In 1993, the NIH, after studying the Pima Indian genetic code, identified a gene that they believe may contribute to insulin resistance and higher rates of diabetes. This gene, called FABP2, produces an intestinal fatty acid binding protein. This protein then produces two amino acids. One of the amino acids, threonine, appears to absorb more fatty acids from fat in a meal. The researchers believe this ultimately leads to higher amounts of fats and fatty acids in the blood and this is what leads to insulin resistance. While the researchers have found these two amino acids may lead to insulin resistance, they have also found a possible third solution to insulin resistance. In the Pima population, there is an enzyme, called protein phosphatase 1, which also appears to cause insulin resistance. Research is still ongoing as to which of the three is most important in fighting insulin resistance among the Pima.

Many researchers agree that our Western lifestyle, in relation to diet and exercise, may have a direct link to some "preventable" diseases, such as heart disease and Type 2 Diabetes, also known as adult onset diabetes. Type 2 Diabetes traditionally did not develop until a person was in their mid-50s. But, this trend is changing, mostly in part to the growing number of overweight and obesity rates. Overweight people are those whose body mass index (BMI) is 25 or greater; while obese people have a BMI of 30 or greater. Obesity is broken down into two categories—obese and extreme or morbidly obese, which has a BMI of 40 or greater. For woman, it is normal to have approximately 25% of body fat and for men to have approximately 17% of body fat. However, being overweight or obese can cause unnecessary stress and strain on your body, can increase a person's resistance to insulin and susceptibility to infections, increase the risk for coronary heart disease and stroke, Type 2 Diabetes, high blood pressure, and kidney disease, as well as other serious health problems which can result in premature deaths.

According to a report by the World Health Organization (WHO), the rates of obesity have risen in every age group in the United States. The report concludes that between 1980 and 2004, the prevalence of obesity in the U.S. has doubled among adults and rose by 17% among children. Overall, approximately 67% of Americans are overweight or obese. African-American women, at 52%, have the highest rates of obesity in the U.S.; while African-American men and white-Americans of both sexes have an approximate 31% obesity rate. In looking at how Americans eat and exercise, 96% stated they could not remember the last time they ate a salad and approximately 40% do not exercise. The lesson is that Americans eat more calories than they burn off by exercising.

The WHO also reported the number of smokers in the U.S. has declined to a record low of 19.8% of our population. This has led to a trend in lower lung cancer cases and deaths. Although this is good news, the WHO also reports 39.5% of adult Americans do not exercise and 29.5% of adult Americans get some exercise. The lack of exercise is directly linked to income, in that more than half of all people living in poverty do not exercise regularly; and poor Latinos are the least likely to exercise. While the average weight of women and children has appeared to stabilize, the rate of obesity among men has continued to rise. Part of this healthier trend for women and children is due to aggressive health-related programs introduced in schools, hospitals, community groups, and churches.

Many researchers believe that Type 2 Diabetes reflects lifestyle issues and is, therefore, a lifestyle disease. In particular, these lifestyle issues reflect an imbalance between calories ingested and calories exerted by physical activity and exercise. A recent article published in Pediatrics showed that more children are eating "fast" foods, which are higher in calories and fats and are less likely to eat balanced meals, which include fresh fruits and vegetables. Also, children and adults are less likely to engage in physical activities and exercise, including the simple task of walking. In another study, there was a direct correlation between the number of hours of television a child watched on a daily basis and the prevalence of obesity. Therefore, the more television was watched, the less exercise and physical activity the child engaged in. According to a report by the National Council of La Raza (NCLR), it was noted that there are three main risk factors for becoming overweight; the first being—genetics, the second being—diminished physical activity, and the third being—greater reliance on high-calorie, high-fat foods associated with poverty and food insecurity.

Unfortunately, this disturbing trend is not limited to the youth of the U.S., but is rapidly becoming a global problem. Recently, *Time Magazine* reported in a series of articles related to obesity in our children and the growing trend around the world. What they found was that as more people adapt the "American, western-style" of eating, more children are experiencing higher rates of obesity. According to a second *Time Magazine* article, "Obesity Goes Global," the U.S. leads the way for industrialized countries with 37% of

American children age 5 through 17 that are overweight or obese, as compared to 20% of European children and 10% of Chinese children. Health ministers fear that obese children will become obese adults. This will eventually lead to higher rates of chronic and debilitating diseases, such as heart disease, hypertension, diabetes, and cancer. According to a Hungarian doctor, 9% of obese children and adolescents have a pre-morbid condition known as "metabolic syndrome." This syndrome, which has elevated of LDL "bad" cholesterol level and elevated blood "sugar" levels, is the precursor to Type 2 Diabetes or adult onset diabetes. Health officials in China believe that if the trends continue, the rate of diabetes among their children and adolescents will double in the next ten years.

In studies by several European organizations, it was found that obesity and growing health problems associated with obesity are not limited to the United States. Because the age-old Mediterranean diet, which included fresh fish, fruits and vegetables, pasta and olive oil, is losing out to the American-style of eating, an increasing number of European adults and children are becoming overweight and obese at an alarming rate. According to doctors at the Rome Federation of Pediatrics, they believe that many Europeans, in general, have lost the healthy eating habits of sitting down with the whole family and eating healthier prepared meals. Many more European adult and children are eating outside of the home, which means more "fast" foods and packaged snack foods. These processed foods are higher in saturated fats, higher in processed sugars, and higher in calories. It was also noted that many more children and adolescents are less physically active, with many physical activity in schools limited, and are spending an average of four to five hours a day on front of a television or on a computer. This "Americanized" style of diet and of lifestyle choices are believed to be the main causes of their country's overweight and obesity problems.

According to the Organization of Economic and Cultural Development (OECD) study, data from 1999–2001 showed the United Kingdom has the second highest percentage of obese adults at 22%, while Spain has 13%, Finland has 11%, Denmark has 10%, and Sweden, France, and Italy all having 9%, as compared to the United States at 31%. In another study on obesity, the International Obesity Task Force (IOTF), which is a number of London-based consumer groups which work in collaboration with the World Health Organization, found disturbing numbers of obesity for European children age 6 to 13 years. The IOTF reported Italy had the highest percentage of obese children at 36%, with Spain not that far behind at 30%, while the United Kingdom has 22%, Denmark, France, and Sweden all having 18%, and Finland has13%, as compared to the U.S. at 15%.

Because of the alarming rate these numbers are growing, many countries are beginning to institute measures in order to combat the medical consequences and long-term costs that are associated with obesity. Sweden has negotiated voluntary restrictions on television advertising aimed at children for "junk" foods, such as snacks and soft drinks; while England is pushing for a ban on this type of advertising during preschool television programs. Italy is looking at several ways to fight their obesity problems; by negotiating with restaurants to reduce the size of portions and by making Friday a day of fasting.

According to a report by The National Institute of Public Health (NIPH), in Mexico two of every three people are either overweight or obese, and many of those die of Type 2 Diabetes or diabetes-related complications. Mexico is now considered to be the "second fattest" country in the world, behind the United States. Over the years, several studies by the Mexican government have shown a rise in the number in the rates of obesity and diabetes; in which the percentage of Mexican women considered to be obese spiking 160% between 1988 and 1999. In 2000, approximately 60% of Mexican men and 64% of Mexican women were considered overweight or obese. As of 2008, a recent study showed that 66% of Mexican men and 71% of Mexican women were obese. A 2002 government study in Mexico City, reported that 30% of Mexican elementary-age school children and 45% of adolescents were overweight or obese.

In the poorest rural areas of Mexico malnutrition is a major concern, with 10 to 12% of the population suffering from malnutrition. However, even in these poor communities, obesity is becoming a growing problem. Many of the poor are turning to the growing availability of the cheap and convenient industrialized processed foods, which in most cases are devoid of nutrients and are calorie dense. In 2000, it was found that among Mexican families of the less wealthy, their children had an increased body weight of 40% and one quarter of the children age five to 11 years were overweight.

With globalization and modernity, the citizens of Mexico are adopting the lifestyle habits of their neighbors to the north—the United States. The traditional healthy diet of Mexicans, which included corn and beans along with fresh fruits and vegetables and the sparingly use of meat and dairy products, is now being replaced by prepared processed foods, made from white flour, saturated fats, and processed sugars. The pinto and black beans, which are nutrient dense foods, are being replaced with processed pasta soups and other microwavable foods. Even the traditional corn tortilla is being replaced with a white flour tortilla and cheap white bread. But Mexico does not import all of its fast foods, as there is an infinite variety of home grown junk food. Although numerous stores and street stands may sell fresh fruits and juices, many sell cookies, snacks, potato chips, and candy. One of the problems Mexico faces is that approximately 80% of schools do not have access to drinking water. Therefore, it is easier for the schools to provide soft drinks. Currently, Mexico comes in second to the U.S. in the amount of soft drinks consumed, with the amount of soft drinks consumed over the last 14 years rising by 60%. The eating habits of Mexicans has totally transformed from healthier traditional foods to convenient processed foods and to the growing number of American "fast" food chains that have spread over the last ten years.

Unfortunately, Mexico also recognizes the other American lifestyle habit that has contributed to their growing obesity problem—a decline in physical activity. Along with modernity, there is no longer the opportunity to burn off the calories that the body takes in. Because of technical advances, the lack of manual labor can be easily seen in the larger cities, and these advances are making their way to the smaller rural communities. Mexico also recognizes that because of technological advances, the lack of health and physical activity in schools has been reduced over the years. In the 2002 study, it was found in elementary schools approximately 32% of children in South Mexico City exercise and 60% of these children are not considered overweight or obese. Mexico recognizes there are not enough physical education programs in the school systems. In 2008, the Mexican Health Secretary began a program with the goal of increasing physical activity among elementary-aged children.

The spike in obesity rates is believed to be the main cause of the rising numbers of those being diagnosed with diabetes, which is estimated to be at approximately 11%. According to the Health Ministry in Mexico, diabetes is now the leading cause of death among Mexican adults. In addition, the diabetes-related diseases can lead to health problems that shorten the life span of Mexicans; with approximately 70,000 dying of diabetes each year. This places a tremendous strain on Mexico's health care system, and currently Mexico is spending the majority of its health care budget on diabetes and diabetes-related diseases.

Health Disparities among Various Groups

In the fifth annual study "F is for Fat: How Obesity Policies Are Failing America, 2008" from the Trust for America's Health (TFAH) and the Robert Wood Johnson Foundation (RWJF), it was found the obesity epidemic our country faces is lowering our productivity and increasing our health care costs. In addition, this report states that more than 25% of adults are obese in 28 states; that obesity rates for adults rose in 37 states and no state showed a decrease in obesity rates; and the number of states in which obesity rose for the third consecutive year was 19 states. Eleven of the 15 states with the highest obesity rates were in the South, in which Mississippi had the highest rate of adult obesity at 31.7% and is also one of the states in which obesity rates have risen for the third consecutive year. It was also reported that obesity and diabetes are linked with poverty levels; in which seven of the 10 highest obesity rates are also in the top 10 for highest poverty rates. What is also disturbing is that with the rise in obesity rates, the rate of Type 2 Diabetes rose in 26 states last year, as well.

In this section, I want to look at one of the most devastating diseases — Diabetes Mellitus or Type 2 Diabetes. Also known as adult onset diabetes, this disease does not discriminate among any one ethnic group, nor does it discriminate based on age or gender. This disease can and will strike any one person, as long as preventative measures and healthcare are not made available. As stated above, there are many causes for one person developing Type 2 Diabetes, from having a gene that predisposes you having the disease to familial inherited prevalence of the disease to poor diet and poor exercise habits. Whatever the cause, diabetes rates for those of minority and/or ethnic populations are at an all time high and are expected to rapidly grow. The prevalence for developing this disease is highest among the following ethnic minorities: Native-Americans, Mexican-Americans, and African-Americans. However, children and adolescents, age 20 years and younger, are one of the fastest growing age groups for developing "diabesity," which is diabetes and obesity.

Native-Americans

Native-American diabetes rates are not as consistent as most ethnic groups. Currently there are more than 560 federally recognized tribes in the United States (U.S.) and approximately 100 other tribes that are recognized by each individual state. Each tribal community has a culture that is unique for their members. This also applies to how each tribal community views health beliefs and health practices. Unfortunately diabetes is not limited to Native Americans in the U.S. Those who are Indigenous Peoples of Canada and Mexico are also finding the rates of diabetes on the rise. Taking into consideration that these two countries also have numerous tribes with cultural beliefs that are vastly different from Native Americans in the U.S., one cannot and must not try to apply one solution to this growing problem among all the Native and Indigenous Peoples of North America. According to medical experts, Native-Americans in the U.S. have the highest rate of diabetes in the world.

According to the Department of Health and Human Services (DHHS), Indian Health Services (IHS), Division of Diabetes Treatment and Prevention, 95% of those Native Americans with diabetes have Type 2 Diabetes. Data from the 2005 database of the Indian Health Service (IHS) estimates the 14.2% of American Indians and Alaskan Natives, age 20 years and older, are diagnosed diabetics who received care from the IHS for this disease. However, after adjusting for age differences among the population, it is actually estimated that 16.5% of the adult population has diagnosed diabetes. According to the National Diabetes Information Clearinghouse (NDIC), this foundation believes that data used to estimate the prevalence of diabetes among Native Americans underestimates the true prevalence of this disease. During a 2002 diabetic screening study in three geographic areas, the NDIC found that between 40% and 70% of Native Americans age 45 to 74 years were found to have diabetes.

According to the DHHS, The Office of Minority Health, on average in 2005 American Indian/Alaska Natives adults are 2.3 times more likely than white adults to be diagnosed with diabetes and in the state of Hawaii; Native Hawaiian adults are 5.7 times more likely than white adults living in Hawaii to be diagnosed with diabetes. The CDC reported that between 1990 and 1998, the rate of diagnosed diabetes in Native Americans age 35 years and younger had increased by 71%, with the greatest number being Native American women. Furthermore, the IHS reports that Native American women age 65 and older have a 25% prevalence rate of being a diagnosed diabetic, as compared to 11.2% of non-Hispanic white women age 65 and older.

The CDC report shows that the diabetes prevalence rate varies widely among Native Americans within the seven geographic regions in the U.S.: Alaska, Great Lakes, Northern Plains, Pacific, Southeast, Southern Plains, and the Southwest, of which the Southeast had the highest prevalence rate of 34.9 per 1,000 adults age 35 years and younger. When looking into specific groups within the Native American population, the prevalence rate is not accurate for all the different groups. In looking at the percent of Native American communities diabetes rates, Alaskan Native adults have the lowest rate of diabetes at 6%; and even this varies for each sub-group. According to the NDIC, among this age 20 and older, Eskimo groups have a prevalence rate of 12.1 per 1,000, Indian groups 24.3 per 1,000, and the Aleut 32.6 per 1,000. The NDIC also reported in their survey that among Navajo adults age 20 and older; 22.9% were diagnosed with diabetes, 14% had a history of diabetes, and 7% were undiagnosed, while the IHS official rate for diabetes among Navajo adults age 45 and older is 40%. Native American adults in southern Arizona have the highest rate of diabetes at 29.3%, with approximately 50% of Pima Indian adults age 30 and 64 having a diagnosis of diabetes. Lastly, the Minnesota Department of Health conducted a population-based study in 2001, which showed that the rate of diabetes among Native Americans in Minnesota and Wisconsin was 600% higher than the rate for non-Hispanic whites in these two states.

This diabetic disparity among Native Americans among the Pima Indians, which was described in the "Causes" section, is a classic example of how devastating diabetes can become. Because of the "thrifty gene" they have higher rates of insulin resistance and diabetes than any other Native American in the U.S. Their rate of diabetes is even higher than their Pima Indian counterparts in Mexico. When researchers visited the Pima Indians in the small rural community in the remote area of the Sierra Madre Mountains in Mexico, they found lower rates of obesity and diabetes. Of those 35 Mexican Pima studied, only 3 were diabetic and, as a whole, the total population was not overweight. They believe that although the Mexican Pima were genetically the same as the Arizona Pima, those in Mexico still lived in the old traditional way, which included a high degree of physical activity and a diet that is lower in fat and higher in starch. According to the National Institute of Diabetes and Digestive and Kidney Diseases (NIDDK), obesity is a major risk factor in the development of diabetes among the Pima Indians. Furthermore, one-half of adult Pima Indians have diabetes and 95% of those with diabetes are overweight.

The American Diabetes Association (ADA) recognizes that diabetes must be recognized and treated in a culturally sensitive way. In addition to trying to bring about legislative changes to combat this disease, they have founded several community-based activities in order to bring about positive change among those in the Native American communities. With the "Awakening the Spirit" advocacy program, on a national and local level, volunteers work to Congress for continual support and funding of grassroots diabetic education programs. The ADA also focuses on providing translator education for Native Americans and translation of terms and concepts of diabetes into the Navajo language. According to the DHHS-IHS, Division of Diabetes Treatment and Prevention, in 1997 Congress recognized this growing diabetes epidemic among Native Americans and established the "Special Diabetes Program for Indians." Currently, this program is trying to make quality diabetes care practices commonplace within Native American communities and their healthcare facilities; with a focus on better health outcomes and better quality of life for those Native Americans with diabetes.

Mexican-Americans

Many medical experts believe because Mexican-Americans share genes with the North American Indigenous Peoples or Native-Americans, this is one reason why Mexican-Americans also have one of the highest diabetes rates. Much like the Native-American population, Hispanic/Latino Americans face the same problems when trying to understand the effects of obesity and diabetes within this ethnic group. The term "Hispanic" refers to those groups of people who trace their ancestry to Mexico, Puerto

Rico, Cuba, Spain, the Spanish-speaking countries of Central or South America, the Dominican Republic or other Spanish cultures, regardless of race; while the term "Latino" includes those people of Latin America descent. In many cases, data is difficult to obtain for all "Hispanics" and, therefore, much of the data that is gathered by various organizations and government agencies tend to focus on the largest population in the United States—Mexican-Americans. Information in this section will include overall general information as it pertains to the Hispanic/Latino population, when available. However, most of this section will focus on the Mexican-Americans and their prevalence rates for obesity and diabetes.

In a 2002 U.S. Census Bureau update, it was reported that Mexican-Americans are the largest Hispanic population in the United States; in which 66.9% of the 37.4 million are of Mexican heritage. The second largest group is the Central and South Americans at 14.3%, followed by Puerto Ricans at 8.6%, and a mixture of other Hispanic heritages not in the above groups, such as Cubans, at 6.5%. Overall, the Hispanic/Latino population in the U.S. has the highest non-insurance rate of any ethnic group in the country. And within this population, according to the US DHHS, Office of Minority Health, Mexican-Americans have the highest uninsured rate among the Hispanic/Latino group at 37%. Although all Hispanic/Latino populations have a higher risk of developing diabetes, Mexican-Americans appear to be more disposed to developing diabetes. Mexican-Americans are 1.9 times more likely to develop diabetes than non-Hispanic whites.

There was also a correlation between diabetes and being overweight and/or obese. Overall, Hispanics/Latinos have the highest overweight and obesity rates in the United States. According to the Heart Disease and Stroke Statistics—2006 Update by the American Heart Association (AHA), approximately 66% of U.S. adults age 20 years and over were overweight; and approximately 31.4% of U.S. adults were obese. According to a 2001-2004 National Health and Nutrition Examination Survey (NHANES), National Center for Health Statistics, 39.6% of Hispanics/Latinos age 18 and older were overweight or obese and 27.5% were obese. The NHANES report also indicated that among Mexican-Americans adults age 20 and older 74.6% of men and 73% of women are overweight or obese; and 29.1% of Mexican-American men and 39.4% of women were obese.

In 2007, the CDC released a report which indicated that, while there has been no statistical change in the number of Americans that are obese, the numbers are still high. The CDC report indicates that 34% of American adults age 20 and over are obese, of which 51% of Mexican-American women age 40-59 years and 37% of Mexican-American women age 60 and over were obese. Obesity is a major contributor to the onset of Type 2 Diabetes, especially among Mexican-American children and adults. According to the National Diabetes Information Clearinghouse (NDIC), the trend for overweight and obesity among Mexican-Americans is rising. Because obesity tends to continue into adulthood, these overweight children are becoming obese adults. The next generation of Mexican-Americans is being diagnosed with Type 2 Diabetes at earlier ages than their non-Hispanic white counterparts.

In the American Heart Association (AHA) 2008 Heart Disease and Stroke Statistics Update, the data collected between the years 1998-2002 showed that diabetes disproportionately affects Hispanics/ Latinos. The AHA also reported that 90-95% of those Hispanic-Americans with diabetes have Type 2 Diabetes or adult onset diabetes. It was reported Hispanics/Latinos are twice as likely to be diagnosed a diabetic than non-Hispanic whites of similar age. The prevalence for diabetes among this ethnic group is as follows: 12.6% are Puerto Rican, 11.9% are Mexican-American, and 8.2% are Cuban. In looking at a breakdown of the rates of diabetes, the AHA reported that the 2005 prevalence of doctor-diagnosed diabetes among Hispanic/Latino adults age 20 and older was 7.3%, the prevalence of undiagnosed diabetes was 2.8%, and the prevalence of pre-diabetes was 27.9%.

According to the 2001-2204 NHANES report, while Hispanics and Latinos are twice as likely to develop diabetes, Mexican-Americans have one of the highest rates. Among Mexican-American adults age 20 years and older, the prevalence for diabetes is 11% of men and 10.9% of women. Within the total population age 20 years and older in which 2.9% of men and 1.9% of women have undiagnosed diabetes; the prevalence of undiagnosed diabetes Mexican-American men is 1.1% and 3.1% for women. However, within the total population age 20 years and older in which 33.8% of men and 21.7% of women are pre-diabetic; the estimated prevalence of pre-diabetes among Mexican-Americans age 20 years and older is 37.5% of men and 22.6% of women.

According the AHA, approximately 65% of those with diabetes, die from complications of the disease, such as heart disease and/or stroke, and not from diabetes mellitus or Type 2 Diabetes. It was also estimated that heart disease death rates among those adults with diabetes was two to four times higher than those adults without diabetes. According to the CDC, in 2003 the prevalence for any type of self-reported cardiovascular condition among those with diabetes among Hispanics age 35 and older was 29.9% for men and 23.7% for women. Other diabetes-related complications occur higher among Hispanics/Latinos. Diabetic retinopathy is a condition in which abnormalities of the blood vessels in the eye cause them to break and/ or leak. If left untreated or if a person with diabetes cannot control their "sugar," this condition can lead to blindness. Unfortunately, the prevalence of diabetic retinopathy among Mexican-Americans is between 32 and 40%. Also, diabetes is the leading cause of end stage renal disease, or kidney failure. Among those with diabetes, Mexican-Americans are 4.5 to 6.6 times more likely to suffer from end stage renal disease.

African-Americans

According to a 2001-2004 report by the NHANES, National Center for Health Statistics, among African-Americans adults age 20 and older 67% of men and 79.6% of women are overweight or obese; and 30.8% of African-American men and 51.1% of African-American women were obese. In 2007, the CDC released a report which indicated that 34% of American adults age 20 and over are obese, of which 53% of non-Hispanic black women age 40-59 years and 61% of non-Hispanic black women age 60 and over were obese.

African-American diabetes rates are also dramatically increasing. According to the NIDDK, approximately 13% of all non-Hispanic blacks have diabetes. In a NIDDK 1976-1980 study, it was reported that for African-American adults age 40 to 74 years the prevalence rate of diabetes was 8.9%; while 12 years later in a 1988-1994 study reported that the prevalence rate of diabetes more than doubled to 18.2%. According to the DHHS, The Office of Minority Health, African-American adults are 1.9 times more likely to be diagnosed with diabetes than non-Hispanic white adults; African-American adults are 1.7 times more likely to be hospitalized than non-Hispanic whites; and 2.2 times more likely to die from diabetes and the complications of diabetes than non-Hispanic whites.

According to the 2001-2204 NHANES report, African-Americans also have one of the highest rates of developing diabetes. Among African-American adults age 20 years and older, the prevalence for diabetes is 10.7% of men and 13.2% of women. Within the total population age 20 years and older in which 3.6% of men and 2% of women have undiagnosed diabetes; the prevalence of undiagnosed diabetes African-American men is 1.7% and 2.3% for women. However, within the total population age 20 years and older in which 33.5% of men and 22.6% of women are pre-diabetic; the estimated prevalence of pre-diabetes among African-Americans age 20 years and older is 23.1% of men and 20.5% of women.

Although African-Americans have one-third more diabetes, their group experiences less Type 1 diabetes and they develop more diabetes complications, such as heart disease, stroke, kidney failure, and blindness. African-Americans are more likely to develop high blood pressure (hypertension) than non-Hispanic whites, but have lower rates of high cholesterol levels than non-Hispanic whites. According to the CDC, in 2003 the prevalence for any type of self-reported cardiovascular condition among those with diabetes among African-Americans age 35 and older was 31.3% for black men and 28.9% for black women. Ischemic stroke, in which an artery to the brain is blocked, is more common in those with diabetes and hypertension; and this risk is more prominent before the age of 55 in blacks, than before the age of 55 in non-Hispanic whites.

Other diabetes-related complications occur in higher rates for African-Americans than in their non-Hispanic/Latino white counterpart. African-Americans are more likely to undergo lower-extremity amputations than non-Hispanic whites or even within the Hispanic/Latino population. African-Americans are also 2.6 to 5.6 times more likely to suffer from diabetes-related end stage renal disease than non-Hispanic whites. Lastly, African-Americans are 40-50% more likely to develop diabetic retinopathy, because of the combined effects of diabetes and hypertension.

Children and Adolescents

The AHA 2008 Update also reported from the CDC's 2005 survey, estimated that more than 9 million children and adolescents, ages 6-19 years old, are considered to be overweight. In addition, this report stated that another 16.5% of children and adolescents, ages 2-19 years, are at risk for becoming overweight.

For ages 2-5 years, the number of overweight pre-school children increased from 10.3% in 1999-2000 to nearly 14% in 2003-2004. Among pre-school children that are overweight, 19.2% are Mexican-American, 13% are non-Hispanic black, and 11.5% are non-Hispanic white. The prevalence of being overweight was highest among Hispanic students, ages 6-19 years, of which 16.8% were overweight, as compared to 16% non-Hispanic blacks and 11.8% non-Hispanic whites. For children ages 6-11 years, the number of overweight children increased from 4% in 1971-1974 to 17.5% in 2001-2004; while for ages 12-19 years, this increased from 6.1% to 17% during the same periods.

According to the ADA, although Type 2 Diabetes can occur in young children, under the age of 20 years, the diabetes trends for this age group in not available. Currently, the diagnosis of Type 2

Diabetes cases in children is considered rare. However, the ADA mentions that this disease is now being diagnosed more frequently than in the past, particularly among American Indians, African Americans, and Hispanic/Latino Americans.

Children now have their own special disease, "diabesity," which is a combination of diabetes and obesity. This is becoming an epidemic among our children. More children are being diagnosed with diabesity at younger ages than before, which is an early sign that they may develop Type 2 Diabetes at an even younger age. Unfortunately, many children are now beginning to experience a higher diagnosis rate of Type 2 Diabetes and this rate is expected to grow rapidly over the coming years. During 2008, there were numerous studies and articles published in relation to this growing health trend among our children. Although those in the medical field, such as physicians, nutritionists, and medical researchers, agree that something needs to be done with this alarming problem among our children, many do not agree with what needs to be done.

According to the American Academy of Pediatrics (AAP), in early 2008 they made the recommendation that statin drugs, used to lower and control cholesterol levels, be given to children as young as two years of age. Because these children had elevated levels and came from families that had a history of abnormally high cholesterol levels, known as hypercholesterolemia. The AAP felt that although this was a desperate and radical approach, that this is a justified attempt to lower the risk of developing heart disease, diabetes, and other diseases that are related to obesity. With the potential to have a record number of children on statin drugs, we need to look at what other alternatives there are for them. Statin drugs are used to control higher cholesterol levels and are at times used in conjunction with other diabetic medications. While, statins are believed to be safe, they are not without risk. Studies have shown that in adults, and in rare cases, statins can cause muscle weakness and kidney problems. There is very limited information as to how statins can affect children. Some doctors see this as a quick fix to address the primary problem—obesity. Many believe that by fixing one problem with a pill, that has no known causes and side effects, you may create other health problems which may then require another pill.

While this problem seems to have no immediate solution, there are issues about obese children that must be addressed. There are many physical and medical problems that they will encounter. According to researchers at Children's Mercy Hospital in Kansas City, who studied obese children and teens, they found obese children have arteries of middle-aged people. The study included 70 children who had an inherited form of familial hypercholesterolemia or were diagnosed with hypercholesterolemia and/or were obese. The arteries of those obese children aged much faster than those of normal-weight counterparts. Using a high-tech ultrasound scan to measure the thickness of the artery wall, the neck arteries had as much plague buildup as a middle-age person in their 40s. This plague buildup can lead to heart attacks and strokes. This study also showed that 75% of those children had advanced vascular ages, especially those with hyperlipidemia or high triglyceride levels, a blood fat.

In a second study, researchers from Cincinnati Children's Hospital were able to confirm that teens and young adults, age range 10 to 24, who are obese or have Type 2 Diabetes showed early signs of heart disease. By using ultrasound imaging the researchers were able to confirm the presence of fatty plaque buildup in the carotid arteries. These arteries, which are found in the neck, carry blood from the heart to the brain. When compared to normal weight youth, those obese and diabetic youth had thicker and stiffer carotid arteries, which are risk factors for heart attack and stroke in adults. This study also found that those obese and diabetic youth were more likely to have high blood pressure and high cholesterol.

In another related study by Australian researchers, they found that obese children are also mostly likely to have enlarged hearts. In looking at the heart, the left atrium is the chamber of the heart where the blood is received from the lungs and sent to the ventricle. Obese children were more likely to have a left atrial size that was significantly larger than in their overweight and normal-weight counterparts. And overweight children had a left atrial size larger than normal-weight children. Those with an enlarged left atrial have a higher risk of developing and dying from heart disease.

All of the above information paints a very bleak picture for our future and the future of our children. However, given the chance to take control of our lives through positive change and by developing healthier choices in both diet and exercise, we can change these poor health trends for the better.

One Family's History of Disease

In the previous section I focused on one of the most devastating diseases, Diabetes Mellitus or Type 2 Diabetes. Also known as adult onset diabetes, this disease has the potential to do a great deal of damage to all of body's major organs and extremities. I choose this specific disease, from the many others that can and do affect many others, because I know firsthand exactly how devastating Type 2 Diabetes can be once it becomes a part of your family's medical history. Not only was my maternal grandmother a Type 2 Diabetic, but my mother along with her fourteen siblings were also Type 2 Diabetics, with five of the fourteen having a dual diagnosis of hypertension or high blood pressure. Also, two of my paternal uncles and one paternal aunt were also Type 2 Diabetics. Recently, my older sister was diagnosed with Type 2 Diabetes. I want to take this opportunity to tell you what diabetes did to my family and why it became important for me to try to gain control of my eating and exercise habits.

Officially, Type 2 Diabetes took a hold of my family in the late 1970s, when my grandmother went in for her second cataract surgery, after she had cataract surgery done several years earlier. Before her surgery, the hospital decided it needed to order a complete blood panel, along with other tests. It was at this point she was told she did not have cataracts, but was actually a Type 2 Diabetic, and as a direct result developed diabetic retinopathy. This was why she was beginning to lose her sight. The uncontrolled "sugar" levels made the blood vessels in her eyes weak and brittle. As they broke, blood and other fluids leaked into the retina and blood leaked into the middle part of her eye in front of her retina. Even though new blood vessels formed, these were just as weak as the older damaged vessels. Over time, this changed her vision and caused her blindness. Until my grandmother showed one of the most serious complications of diabetes, she was unaware that she was a diabetic. For years she missed all of the early signs of this disease. Earlier diagnosis may have delayed her blindness or even may have prevented her blindness.

At the time of my grandmother's death, this disease had taken its toll on her body. She was blind, had an enlarged heart, her circulatory system in her feet and legs were in failure, her kidney was damaged and going into failure, and she had undergone a leg amputation. When she entered the hospital just before Mother's Day in 1993, she believed that she had a minor infection at the tip her toes. After an examination, the doctors called for an amputation of her foot, just below her ankle. Then during the surgery, they found that the circulatory problem in her foot was, in fact, much more damaging to her entire leg. The decision was made to amputate her leg, just below her knee. Sadly, she never recovered from the surgery. So traumatized by the surgery, she could only lie in a hospital bed in a semi-comatose state. Then five days before her birthday, her system began to shut down, she suffered a major heart attack and died alone in a cold hospital bed, with no family present. Ironically, she was laid to rest on her birthday.

The next victim of this disease was my mother's older sister. During the early 1980s, she was diagnosed a Type 2 Diabetic after she had experienced several severe heart problems. She had undergone several bypass heart surgeries to resolve this problem of blocked arteries. Because she could not control her weight or her "sugar" levels and did not know enough about diet and exercise, she was unable to control either disease. She also had a partial leg amputation and was looking at some rapid deterioration of her other leg. A few years after the death of her mother, my grandmother, my aunt suffered a near fatal stroke and lost her ability to speak. After she was stabilized, she was moved into a long-term care facility. During her stay at the facility she was never able to regain her ability to communicate, she began to suffer seizures, and was entirely bedridden. These seizures, which occurred several times a week, kept her very weak. Then almost five and a half years later, during one of the seizures she passed away.

Both of the long and lingering deaths of my aunt and my grandmother put a great deal of fear into my mother and what the future as a diabetic held for her. My mother was diagnosed a diabetic in May 1985, just two months before her 51st birthday. Since the mid-1960s, my mother had always struggled with her weight. She would go on "fad" diets of the 60s, 70s, and through part of the 80s. Because of her issues with her weight, once her mother was diagnosed with diabetes, she always felt she would be diagnosed with diabetes, as well. Needless to say, she was stricken with the news that she was in fact a diabetic. She began a program to lose weight, to keep the weight off, to try to eat healthier, and to exercise. Unfortunately, what she did not know is that she was most likely a diabetic since the mid-1960s. This caused a lot of damage to her body that she was not aware of.

Although, she believed she was able to "control" her disease, she was not savvy enough to understand the complexities of food and how it actually affected your body. The only "diet tricks" she remembered were her rules from some of her most successful diets, such as Weight Watchers and the grapefruit diet. In total, she lost about 90 to 95 pounds and kept it off, but she still had some problems controlling all of her blood glucose levels. While her fasting glucose levels were always within excellent range, her A1C levels were always too high, from 8% to as high as 11%. She failed to understand how and why this specific number was important in relation to her blood sugar. She also did not fully understand how it affected the progression of the disease. Her fear of her doctor, as an authority figure, made her fearful to question the test results or even ask him what they meant. She was unable to ask the important questions regarding her health. Her doctors made the assumption that because she was not asking certain questions, she fully understood what they were telling her. Although she had the determination to try to overcome her diagnosis, she did not possess the health literacy needed to control the disease at an earlier point in her life.

During the last five years of her life when I helped her with her doctors' appointments and helped to guide her in her dietary choices, she was able to gain better control and her A1C went down to 7.1%. Although, she also had developed diabetic retinopathy, she was able to catch it earlier, keep her "sugar" levels under better control, and with the advancement of eye procedures, she was able to keep her sight. The last two and a half years of her life, she actually showed progress and even some reversal of the damage, passed her eye tests, and was surgery free. She believed she was on her way to beating this disease because she was continually getting good feedback from all of her doctors concerning her test results. What she did not know was that her diabetes had weakened her heart and she suffered a "silent" heart attack in November 2005, which caused her heart to become even more fragile. After a nearly 21 year battle with Type 2 Diabetes, my mother passed away suddenly in January 2006. Fortunately, she died instantly from a stroke, caused by cardiovascular heart disease, a common complication of diabetes.

In November 2003, my older sister called me with the sad news that she had been diagnosed a Type 2 Diabetic. She had beaten our mother's diagnosis by about one and half years, being diagnosed three months before her 49th birthday. Although she had not been feeling well over the past several years, she feared the knowledge of having this disease and never went in to the doctor. In the back of her mind she knew that because her weight problems mirrored our mother's, she would become a diabetic. She took a "what you don't know—can't hurt you" approach to her health. At only 4 feet 11 inches, she was slightly over 200 pounds. She told me her cholesterol was over 400 points and her blood glucose levels placed her in the diagnosable category of a Type 2 Diabetic. Needless to say, I was shocked at how high her numbers were, but not surprised at her diagnosis. Her doctor told her had she not come in when she did, she would most likely have had a stroke and could have gone into a diabetic coma or died. This put the fear into her, and she called me for advice about her "diet." Because our mother was doing better following my rules, she wanted to know what advice I gave her. So I sent her the basic information (that is included in this book) and over the next six months she dropped about 75 pounds and her blood glucose levels also improved. To date her blood glucose levels are all within normal range. In her semi-annual checkup in the spring 2009, her A1C level was 6.1%, which is normal for a diabetic. Her doctor even told her that as long as she stays on her diabetic medication and controls her glucose levels, she is technically "no longer a diabetic." Fortunately, she realizes that she will always be a Type 2 Diabetic and works every day to control her disease.

A secondary problem that my sister has is bi-lateral keratoconus, which was diagnosed about twenty years earlier. Although, this eye disease is not directly related to her diabetes, having diabetes does not help this condition. The keratoconus, which is causing both of her corneas to become cone-shaped, interferes with her ability to see clearly. Over the years her eyesight has steadily worsened; while her prescription contacts have become stronger. Without her special contacts needed for this eye condition, she is very close to being legally blind. Unfortunately, she may in the future need a double cornea transplant or run the risk of going blind. Because she is a diabetic, one cannot be sure if she will be a viable candidate for this type of surgery.

The last family member I wish to discuss is my paternal uncle, my father's older brother. For many years he had been in complete denial about the severity of his diagnosis of Type 2 Diabetes. He relied on home remedies to counter any of the symptoms of diabetes. My mother tried to convince him to do the right things, such as lose weight, eat healthier foods, stop his occasional drinking, and take his medication. In October 1999, he was taken to the emergency room, with severe chest pain. Thinking he was having a massive heart attack, he was admitted immediately. Upon his admission, it was found that his blood "sugar," among other levels, was extremely elevated. After stabilizing his condition and running more tests, it was discovered that he was not having a heart attack. His vital organs were in the process of shutting down. He was prepared for emergency surgery. It was found that his pancreas was severely damaged and surgeons had to remove two-thirds of it. Although, he almost died, he managed to survive the surgery. His road to recovery will always be a hard road to travel, because there is no end. He now has to take insulin injections several times a day. If he forgets or does not take them on time, he begins to look disoriented and has something which resembles a seizure. Multiple daily insulin injections are what he will need to do for the rest of his life in order to control his diabetes.

Many would think that these examples are extreme cases within one family of what adult diabetics may face. Because my grandmother, my mother, and my aunt did not know enough about their disease and their prognosis once diagnosed, they were placed at a severe disadvantage to make the necessary healthy changes in their lives. Although they would listen to their doctors explain what they needed to do, they dare not ask HOW they were to go about making the necessary changes in their lives. They were given pieces of paper and brochures that talked about carbohydrates, proteins, and other things in foods and food groups, but never fully understood what these meant and how these things that made up the foods they ate actually affected their blood glucose levels or their bodies. They were neither health literate nor food literate and failed to recognize the importance of diet and exercise, which allowed this disease to progress to a life threatening and, ultimately, a life ending stage. Fortunately for my sister, she is willing to listen to her doctor, ask questions of her doctor, and follow through on the things, such as dietary changes, staying on her medication, keeping routine doctor appointments and blood glucose tests, which will lead her to making better health decisions. As for my uncle, it is up to his children to ensure that he understands and follows the directions of his doctors. After almost dying, he is now more receptive to what his doctors say about his health, especially about his diagnosis as a Type 2 Diabetic.

In the end, what I hope this book to accomplish is for people to get a better understanding of the importance of healthy eating, exercise, and health literacy. With these tools, many will be better equipped to make "healthier" choices for themselves and their family. While it is comforting to think that a "bigger" entity will come in and enact policies that will make this easier for us, we as individuals must take the personal responsibility to understand how our nutritional and other health-related decisions affect us and, more importantly, our children. We need to become health literate, so that we understand why our doctor gives us specific instructions, orders certain tests, and orders specific prescription medications. We need to become our own health advocate in our lives especially when making health-related decisions.

1

The Beginning of Our Personal Journey

Natalia—My Journey

E very person's journey has a beginning. This is mine. In August 1999, I enrolled in a Psychology Behavior Modification class. At the time, I did not realize how this one course would forever change my dietary habits and outlook on foods. Part of this course required us, as students, to pick a bad behavior that we wanted to extinguish and replace it with a good behavior. Of course, I thought I would kill two birds with one stone and made what I believed was a "safe" easy to implement choice of losing a few pounds. For the semester, I decided to monitor my diet, by removing and limiting all "high fat" "high sugar" foods, such as pastries, and adding a formal exercise program into my personal experiment. But first, the instructor for the course required all students that had elected weight loss/exercise programs as part of the experiment to first get a complete physical, to ensure that the dietary and/or physical exercise changes we had chosen would be safe and were also approved by a physician.

I'm the first to admit, my initial incentive was purely one of vanity, since I believed that I was slightly overweight. About three months shy of age 42, standing at 5 feet 1½ inches, and approximately 138 pounds, I was at my heaviest weight in my entire life. Even at age 19 and nine months pregnant, I was only 128 pounds. Looking at my current weight made me feel like I had lost control. I also had a secondary incentive to lose and control my weight, which in reality should have been my only motivating factor. Type 2 Diabetes runs on both my maternal and paternal sides of my family. My maternal grandmother died of complications of diabetes in July 1993 and my mother was diagnosed with diabetes at shortly before age 51. Most people, not knowing about my family history, could not understand why I felt so badly about being a "little heavy." They thought I was being silly to concentrate so much on my "non-problem" of being almost 140 pounds and wanting to lose weight.

After completing my blood work and getting my test results that fall, I was shocked to learn that my triglycerides were off the chart, slightly over 1,000. The normal level should be below 150 and the borderline high levels are 150−199. Although, all of my other blood glucose levels were within acceptable normal ranges, my doctor was not happy and immediately placed me on a generic lopid, Gemfibrozil, which is in the cholesterol-lowering class of fibrates and related to fenofibrates and statins. Along with my new medication, he encouraged me to continue with the weight loss/exercise program. By the end of the course, I lost twelve pounds, although my triglycerides were still high at around 800. Although, my doctor was not completely happy, he advised me to continue with my new medication. Unfortunately this continued for two years, with my triglycerides slowly decreasing. While on Gemfibrozil, the lowest my triglycerides ever went down to was a little over 500 during the spring of 2001.

Then in the fall 2001 a different doctor, within the same physician's association, took me on as a patient. Not happy with my still high triglycerides test results, he decided to take me off Gemfibrozil and placed me on Tricor. This was the newest fenofibrate, which showed promise in lowering both high triglycerides and high cholesterol. Although I knew there were some adverse side effects and, in some cases, severe complications with Tricor, I knew I needed to lower my triglycerides. During the first weeks after starting Tricor, I began to have migraines. The doctor advised me to give my body time to adjust to the new medication, and if I still had problems after the second month, then he would change my medication or lower the dose. For the first six weeks, I suffered from extreme migraines to, thankfully, mild migraines, then to an occasional migraine. I stayed on Tricor for a little over two years and I could not get my triglycerides below 400. I was still working to control my weight. Along with the headaches, I had erratic mood swings and began to experience a "tingly" sensation and some muscle pain throughout my legs, and especially my lower arms and fingers. I was also experiencing constant neck pain, which I contributed to the stress I felt I was under with my medical condition.

I have to point out that I was not a passive dieter during these four years. I tried every diet trick possible, "low-fat," "no-fat," "sugar-free," "counting calories," "counting carbohydrates," etc. No matter what I tried, my weight would level off for a period of time, but my triglycerides still remained high and I would regain some weight, as well. Then in August 2003, after returning home from summer vacation, I went in for my annual physical and, once again, routine blood tests were ordered. I state routine, because in my case I was getting blood tests every six months. I knew that I had not maintained a "proper" diet while camping during the summer. I knew that I had eaten a diet higher in carbohydrates than was wise, although cooking rice dishes over a campfire is faster and easier, but in the end not healthier. I worked extra hard to stay on a better diet when I returned home. Once at home, my husband decided to go to a more indigenous way of eating, since we are both of Native American descent. He explored the foods that both our peoples ate and started to incorporate these foods into our diets. For example, we began to eat more blueberries, wild rice, corn-based products, beans, etc. We also limited the amount of processed foods and began to eat more homemade meals.

As I expected, the August tests results showed not only were my triglycerides still high, but what surprised me was they were the highest ever, at slightly over 1,200. I now had a secondary problem to deal with. My cholesterol was over 250. Normal total cholesterol should be below 200, borderline high is 200-239, and high cholesterol is 240 and above. To make matters worse, my weight had gone back to 138 pounds. I could not believe that all my "dieting," exercise, and staying on medication was having little to no effect. It was not until the beginning of November that my doctor had his assistant call me to inform me of my test results and that he wanted to add the newest statin medication on the market, the super-statin Crestor. Crestor was estimated to be two to three times more potent than Lipitor and up to six times more potent than Zocor. According to the assistant, Crestor was hailed as the newest wonder drug to reduce both triglycerides and cholesterol. I was more angry than devastated about the test results for two reasons. First, that it took almost three months for my doctor's office to notify me of the results and second, that my doctor wanted to add another stronger drug without any type of consultation.

Although I followed my doctors' advice in the past, I was feeling a mixture of emotions. I felt angry, because my doctor decided to just "casually" add another new drug without first discussing this drug with me. I felt disappointed, because another drug was being added, along with one that obviously was not working for me. I felt scared and concerned, because I had heard some patients had suffered severe complications, such as extreme muscle weakness, associated with some drugs in the statin class, such as Baycol. I was also disillusioned because I thought I was a failure and that I was going to follow in my family's footsteps and eventually be diagnosed a diabetic before age 50. So instead of taking his decision lying down, I requested another test to re-verify the results, before going ahead with the addition of Crestor. I knew that I had tried to be more conscious of my eating habits since returning home from vacation and had actually lost a few pounds, so I hoped that my November tests would prove to be better.

However, what I mostly felt like was an invisible patient. I believed my doctors were not listening to what I perceived could be a causal factor to my ongoing problem. Because my mother and older sister had gone into early menopause, 36 years of age and 39 years of age, respectively, I was convinced that I went into perimenopause at age 40. I had begun experiencing hot flashes, insomnia, and forgetfulness. I started taking 80 mg of standardized black cohosh extract daily, which helped to ease the symptoms. But, I now believe the black cohosh helped to mask my menopause symptoms. My doctors believed I was too young, even with my family history, to be in perimenopause. My FSH (follicle-stimulating hormone) test did not indicate I was in perimenopause and my doctors did not know whether or not the black cohosh I was taking could alter or affect the test results. The FSH test is now believed to be somewhat unreliable in determining whether or not a woman is in menopause. Besides, my doctors were, by their own admission, not very informed about herbal remedies in general. So for me, this was troubling they would casually overlook this as a secondary diagnosis. From what I had read, once a woman starts to go through the stages of menopause, changes in the body and body chemistry will occur that can include weight gain, increased cholesterol, and elevated blood sugar levels. My doctors did not consider the possibility that I could be in perimenopause and this condition could be causing my increased cholesterol and high tri levels and therefore not properly treating my condition.

In the meantime my husband, who was very supportive, got really proactive and found different and some conflicting evidence about the diet plans that I had tried to follow and even the prescription drugs being recommended for me. But the thing we found to be the most discouraging, and what changed our opinion the most was that Crestor, a super-statin, was in the same class as Baycol. I was deeply concerned that I would experience adverse side effects and complications with Crestor, because of my bad experience with Tricor. I researched the available information about Crestor in the *Physicians' Desk Reference 2004* and found the PDR as well as other sources stated that statins and fenofibrates should never be combined, as this could increase the chances of severe complications. A doctor should only under extreme circumstances combine fenofibrates and statins. I did not want to be an extreme case. The PDR went on to state that if fenofibrates do not get the desired results in three to six months then other alternatives should be looked into. My doctors kept me on this class of drugs for over four years.

Through his research, my husband found a natural alternative in pantethine, a vitamin B5 derivative. Multiple studies have shown that pantethine helps to reduce serum triglycerides, total cholesterol and low-density lipoprotein (LDL) or "bad" cholesterol levels, while increasing high-density lipoprotein (HDL) or "good" cholesterol levels in virtually every class of patient. My husband knew that many herbalists believe milk thistle extract helps to promote a healthy liver, which is the organ responsible for changing fats eaten in the diet to types of fat that can be stored and used by the body. Obviously, my liver was not healthy because my triglycerides were so off the charts. Lastly, both fenofibrates and statins block the manufacture of coenzyme Q10 (CoQ10). In some cases, low levels of CoQ10 can cause a predisposition to developing heart disease and muscle-wasting diseases. So in addition to trying to develop a better dietary plan the both of us could follow, my husband and I decided that I would stop taking prescription medication and try the natural supplements for a short period of time to see if I could get better results. So I started taking pantethine, milk thistle, and CoQ10.

My husband then concentrated on perfecting "Natalia's diet" and found different and better ways to prepare foods, foods that would decrease triglycerides and cholesterol naturally. We looked at different foods that we both enjoyed eating and began to practice the many ways of preparing these foods in a healthier manner. What aided me the most was a book that helped me to understand how to incorporate the foods we ate traditionally with foods that we are supposed to eat to maintain a healthier lifestyle. *Super Foods Rx: Fourteen Foods That Will Change Your Life*, by Dr. Steven Pratt helped me to put in perspective how the foods of our traditions and cultures could be incorporated into our daily eating habits. It explained why and how different foods promoted a healthier lifestyle and how they had preventative qualities against some diseases and illnesses.

As I said earlier, in November 2003, I ordered new test results. My test results showed my triglycerides were 919 and total cholesterol 265. In March 2004 after just four months on my new regimen, my test results showed my triglycerides were 718 (a 22% decrease) and my total cholesterol 247 (a 7% decrease). Then in August 2004, my husband and I found a new doctor. After ordering blood tests as part of our annual physical examination, my test results showed my triglycerides dropped to 414 (an additional 41% decrease) and my total cholesterol 209 (an additional 15% decrease). I also went from 138 pounds to 122 pounds in weight. Basically, changes in my eating plan gave me the same results, as the prescription medications the doctors had prescribed. Although my doctor was concerned that my levels were still elevated, he was somewhat pleased to find that in approximately nine months, my total tri level decreased 55% and my total cholesterol level decreased 21%. After discussing my dietary and exercise plan with him, he felt I would be able to continue with my changes, as long as I kept him informed of any problems or changes and, more importantly, continued to get blood tests every three months.

He also confirmed that I was in perimenopause and that my current diet and exercise plan would be beneficial. Because I was apprehensive about hormone replacement therapy, I added soy supplement to help with my increasing night sweats and hot flashes. But, I needed to be careful with the soy supplement. Some dieticians do not condone the use of soy supplements. They instead prefer soy intake in its whole natural states, such as soymilk, soybeans, and other soy-based products, in order to properly control age-related problems associated with menopause. Although, soy supplements can help with most menopause symptoms, some dieticians believe these supplements cannot be adequately standardized. Also, because the results of multiple studies vary, one should use soy supplements carefully and discontinue them if you find them problematic.

In September 2005, with my weight still under control, my test results showed my cholesterol dropped to a perfect 174 (an additional decrease of 17%) for an overall decrease of 34%, and my HDL "good" cholesterol and LDL "bad" cholesterol were also within the optimal ranges. Although, my triglycerides were 532, a disappointing 29% increase, I have still maintained an overall 42% decrease from my original starting point of 919. Because these mixed results confused my doctor, he suggested another cause could be part of my ongoing problem. He believed that I could have hypothyroidism, a less diagnosed illness in women within my age group. Because I am proactive when it comes to my health, I began to research this particular illness along with other related conditions.

Hypothyroidism is simply an under active thyroid. It affects mostly women between the ages of 35 to 50. Because some of the hypothyroidism symptoms can be mistaken for menopause symptoms, it is harder to detect. The standard TSH—thyroid stimulating hormone—test has a wide range of .5 to 5.0 and therefore may not recognize a struggling thyroid problem in perimenopausal women. When you have low thyroid hormones, the liver makes fewer LDL receptors. These receptors help to remove the "bad" LDL cholesterol from the blood, so hypothyroidism may lead to an increase in your cholesterol levels, in your triglyceride levels, or both. Although, several years earlier I had tested negative for a thyroid condition, I agreed with my doctor's suspicions that this could be one of the contributing factors in my battle with my high triglycerides.

While researching hypothyroidism, I also found a condition—estrogen dominance—that is linked to perimenopause and hypothyroidism. This condition can lead to an imbalance of progesterone and estrogen. When this imbalance occurs, the estrogen blocks the action of the thyroid hormone, making the thyroid hormone ineffective. Although the thyroid is producing normal amounts of the hormone, symptoms of hypothyroidism may appear. Basically, estrogen dominance does not allow the liver to convert T4s—thyroxine—into the necessary T3s—triiodothyronine.

Although small amounts of T3 are present your body, this active hormone still has a significant impact on your metabolism and both T4 and T3 are needed to regulate body functions. Estrogen dominance has similar symptoms of both perimenopause and hypothyroidism, which can further complicate an accurate diagnosis.

Because soy isoflavones and black cohosh can have an estrogen-like effect on your body, these supplements may unintentionally help to create a progesterone-estrogen imbalance. My next step was to look at what changes I made during the last year, since I had been able to successfully reduce both my cholesterol and triglyceride levels for the last two years. I knew taking black cohosh for almost five years did not seem to interfere with my ability to lower both levels. The only recent change I made during the past year was the addition of the soy supplement. I then decided to research soy and possible thyroid problems and found information that indicated that the isoflavones in soy supplements act as an inhibitor of thyroid peroxidase, which makes T3 and T4. So I decided to remove the soy supplement and made a stronger commitment to add real soy products into my diet. Although, I was not happy that my night sweats and hot flashes might return, I realized it was important to control my triglyceride levels and try other natural and herbal alternatives, such as vitex (chaste tree) extract or tea, for hot flashes. I tried several different herbal supplements in order to relieve hot flashes. Although these seemed to have a mild effect at relieving some of the symptoms, they were not wholly successful.

In early January 2006, my TSH and full panel lipid blood tests were completed. My TSH results were again within the normal range at 2.66. My total cholesterol level was slightly elevated at 236. Although, I know that studies have shown that total cholesterol levels can rise slightly during the winter months. However, my HDL "good" cholesterol increased and my LDL "bad" cholesterol remained within the optimal range. My triglyceride level was 393, for a significant decrease of 26.2% from my September 2005 level. This is the lowest they have been in over five years. My doctor recommended that I try to adhere more closely to my dietary and exercise plans. Several factors caused me to not follow my plans better, one completely justifiable. In October I had minor out-patient surgery, which caused me to focus less on exercising and more on "taking it easy" to recover.

Also, I admit that I went "off" my healthy way of eating a few times during November and December, while I was "recovering" from the surgery. I know I ate more pork products, in the red and green chili stews, and white flour breads while away from home visiting friends during the holidays. Also, I went overboard with the some of my favorite "comfort" foods, such as tortilla chips, and did not take the time to exercise daily. This is something that I was aware of and I should have tried harder to control. Regardless of this small setback, the fact that my triglycerides decreased made me committed to the way I had been eating and exercising. Unfortunately, the incoming year brought about the beginning of a series of major setbacks that ultimately affected my physical and emotional well-being in what I call—the bump in the road of my journey.

The Bump in the Road of My Journey

First, in late January 2006, my mother passed away suddenly from a stroke. Apparently, she had suffered a "silent" stroke during the fall 2005, which damaged her heart. One can only accept the fact that the diabetes had done enough damage in the twenty plus years before her diagnosis in 1985. Also because she took care of herself since her diagnosis, she actually extended the quality of her life. I believe that without her dedication to fighting her disease and the interventions I took, she would not have lived as long as she had. Or even as pain free and virtually complication free. Sometimes one can only do the best they can and make the best decisions and choices with the information they are given. Although, I feel that she left us far too soon, at least she went the way she wanted. She did not suffer the way her mother and sister suffered. Shortly after her death, my father's eight year battle with prostate cancer took a turn for the worse. The cancer spread to his spine and his prognosis was not good. During the spring and summer, he underwent radiation and chemotherapy treatment to prevent the cancer from spreading rapidly. Since my two sisters lived in another state, all the arrangements for his treatment and care became my responsibility.

In January of 2007, almost one year to the day my mother passed away, we received the news that the cancer had spread to his brain and he was given eight weeks to live. He began a series of intensive radiation treatments to help ease the pain of the tumor in his brain. After the treatments ended, I cared for my father in my home, with the wonderful and supportive assistance of hospice care. In March 2007, thirteen months after my mother passed away, my father died. During this time I was on an emotional rollercoaster and not taking very good care of myself. I knew that I had neglected taking care of myself, in order to take care of both my parents. I was in denial about my own health needs.

In May 2007, I went in for an exam and blood tests. I was not feeling well, I was feeling more fatigued than usual, the pain from the "stress" I was feeling was more constant and radiated throughout my body, and wanted to ease some of the anxiety and depression I was feeling. This was a very stressful time, as I was in the process of settling my father's estate, paying outstanding hospital bills he had incurred, and trying to prepare for a summer vacation. But this proved to be another stressor that I did not need at the time. When my test results came in, my triglycerides were 463, which was slightly higher than in January, and my total cholesterol went up 8 points to 244. Although my doctor was not happy, he stated that maybe I needed to take some time to regroup, since the death of both my parents caused an enormous amount of undue stress. He offered to prescribe an anti-depressant, but of course I declined because I was a strong person and did not need the "help." He stated that he wanted me to have blood tests in December, to ensure that I would be given the time to de-stress and focus on my ability to get back to the point I was in January. I went on vacation with the purpose of tackling my setback.

In early December of 2007, I went for my annual exam with

the usual blood tests to check my blood serum levels. Needless to say, I knew with all the stress that I was under that they would not be good. After all, my emotional state was still fragile with the loss of my parents. Also, I had gained about eight pounds and was up to 130 pounds. But, I was not fully prepared for how bad the news would prove to be and how elevated some of the levels were. My triglycerides nearly doubled to 903 and my total cholesterol rose 20 more points to 264. I was so devastated by the news that I actually broke down and cried in his office. I told the doctor that since the death of my parents, I had been overly emotional and this was causing tremendous physical pain. I believed that it was pain caused by the stress in my life. But, my husband quickly interceded and stated that my pain had actually started a few years before my mother passed away. I was just unaware of how often I would complain about being in pain. Because my husband had a suspicion that I had fibromyalgia, because of where the pain was and how the pain radiated, he told our doctor about his suspicions. I then agreed with the doctor's recommendation to begin taking a mild anti-depressant to help me through this difficult time.

Being more determined than I gave him credit for, he took this opportunity and convinced me to try the starting dosage of Lipitor for a while to see if I could get control of my levels. I agreed and just before Christmas I started to take these new prescriptions. With the promise of a six-week complete blood workup and follow-up exam, I strictly followed my rules and made time to exercise every day. The blood tests my doctor ordered for me, included tests to rule out inflammation. Because he could not make the diagnosis of fibromyalgia, he needed to first make sure that my pain was not caused by other conditions, such as arthritis. Two weeks before my exam, I went for the blood test. When I went in to get the results, during the third week of January 2008, I could not believe the difference. In six weeks, I lost six pounds and was down to 124 pounds. So I knew my tests results were going to be better. However, I did not realize how much better they would be. My blood work showed that my triglycerides were 204 and my total cholesterol was within the normal range at 171. With the help of the starting dose of Liptor, I had finally found the hope in doctors and in prescription medications that I had lost many years earlier.

There was also more good news. All my other blood levels were normal and there was no indication of inflammation. By first ruling out the usual causes of pain, he could now make a referral to a rheumatologist. In the meantime, I started to look into what having fibromyalgia meant and what I could expect from a diagnosis of this condition. In researching this condition, I found that the type of pain that I was experiencing had actually started much earlier. But, I had probably dismissed the pain as "just stress" and being in "stressful" situations. This then led me to an awakening of sorts. I linked the muscle pain, in particular the areas of where I had been feeling the pain, to the strange sensations I was feeling in November 2003, while on fenofibrates and statin drugs. Because my previous doctors at the time were not listening to my complaints about the strange sensations and muscle pain throughout my body, they probably missed the early symptoms of fibromyalgia. The literature on statins and statin-related drugs show that one of the extreme side effects is the possibility of muscle pain and aches. So I simply assumed that the statins were the cause of my problems in my arms and legs. This revelation gave me hope that I would finally find the correct road on my journey to health.

In late April 2008, my rheumatologist confirmed my diagnosis of fibromyalgia, which is a chronic condition that is characterized by widespread muscle pain and fatigue. Unfortunately, there are no tests or x-rays that can confirm this condition. However, there are certain criteria used to make this diagnosis. There are tender points on the body, when pressure is applied, which can assist in a proper diagnosis of this condition. However, in a study released in 2008, it was found that patients with fibromyalgia have abnormal blood flow in the brain. Researchers using a brain imaging technique, the single photon emission computed tomography (SPECT), found abnormalities in blood flow. This abnormality, called a brain perfusion, was either below normal or above normal in those that suffered from the pain of fibromyalgia. The level of abnormality was also linked to the severity of pain, disability, anxiety, and depression a person with fibromyalgia felt. Fibromyalgia is on its way to being recognized as a "real medical disease" and not just an "invisible condition."

During the months of March through June 2008, my husband and I made the move to Albuquerque, New Mexico. So I have added relocating into a new home in a new city to the stress I have been under these past two and a half years. However, for both my husband and me, this move was good stress, not bad stress. Moving to Albuquerque felt right at the time and has proven to be a good decision. After enduring a stressful three years, I am still working on controlling my cholesterol and triglyceride levels. For the past year, I have been taking my "starting" dose of Lipitor, as my old doctor did not feel the need to increase the dosage. When I go to my new doctor, I hope that I will find a partner in my journey to control my blood levels and to a keep my on the road to a healthy life. This is why I state it is important to recognize changes in your life will always be ongoing. As for myself, I will continue to be health literate by researching health-related concerns and by continuing to make changes in my health plan. Once again, I have the confidence to continue "my journey" to healthy living.

Kip—My Husband's Journey

My husband's journey began when he tried to understand and help me control my multiple health conditions—both high triglycerides and cholesterol and my entering perimenopause. After all, partners are supposed to support each other through whatever one encounters and he did not want me to be left to do this alone. Although my journey officially began in August 1999, he did not realize that his journey to healthy eating should have begun in the mid 1990s when he was diagnosed with adult onset asthma. Unfortunately, since his diagnosis, his asthma problems were steadily growing worse, with more severe attacks increasing every year. He had resolved himself to the idea that, for the rest of his life, he would be fighting a continuous battle to control his asthma.

His doctors were able to find the environmental factors, such as high ozone level days and plant-based allergies. These conditions triggered his seasonal allergies and would therefore lead to higher risks of "bad" asthma days. He fought these daily and seasonal battles for about seven years before he realized that he needed to be more proactive about this condition. He could not simply rely on his medication to help him control his asthma. He started to try other natural alternative remedies to control his condition. He noticed that whenever he ate hot, spicy foods, such as hot peppers or a bowl of green chili stew, this would help break up the mucus and actually help him to breath. Hot peppers contain capsicum, which gives the pepper its intense spicy hot flavor. In my husband's case, capsicum helps reduce the severity of an asthma attack.

As he began to read more about the healthier ways for me to gain control of my problems, he realized that his own way of eating could be improved as he believed he was slightly overweight, at 228 pounds. Also, he felt that his ongoing weight problem worsened his asthma. So, he felt that finding a way to eat healthier would be beneficial for both of us. He believed that his one and only downfall to eating healthy was his penchant for anything sweet. He realized he always had something sweet to eat with his morning, afternoon, and evening coffee, whether it was store bought or homemade. Even his "adopted" family from a Native American pueblo near Albuquerque knew this was his weakness. As a running joke, they had even given him what they called an "Indian" nickname of "Cookie Monster." During their traditional feast days, they would jokingly tell him that they had to double the recipes for their cookies because they knew he would be coming over to visit. So he knew that this was one area that he needed to control not only for himself, but for me as well.

He knew that if he ate healthier, he would not only be supporting my dietary changes, he could lose weight as well. During the process of trying newer improved ways of eating, he managed to lose some weight. Despite his dieting, he never went below 215 pounds and he could not keep the weight off. His weight spiraled between 215 to 225 pounds. During the fall of 2003, for the first time in his life his cholesterol went above the normal range and was over 210. This, along with his growing asthma problems, did not discourage his resolve to find the answers we both needed. To the contrary, this only made him more determined to find the solution to both our problems.

Because Kip has a doctoral degree in anthropology, he decided to look back at our ancient traditional indigenous ways of eating and to try to incorporate those ways into a normal health plan. He found that we already ate a lot of healthy foods, such as corn tortillas, low saturated fat foods, like poultry, and lots fresh fruits and vegetables. Then, while browsing one day at a local bookstore, I found the 14 Super Foods book and jokingly stated that we should follow this plan. After reviewing this book, he suggested that I should use it as a guide for how we needed to improve what we ate. It would also give me the background to understand the nutritional values of certain foods and why they are important and should be included in our diet. Because this book stated that many of the foods you eat should be whole foods, we both agreed that for our way of eating this could be hard to incorporate into a daily eating plan. Although, we believed that we already incorporated a lot of whole foods in our diet, we did not think that we could eat entirely whole food. So we agreed that we needed to blend all of our knowledge on the foods we ate with the basic ideas of the book and develop our own rules of eating and shopping (see Chapter Three). This needed to be done in order to make the changes and to follow this new healthy way of eating.

At the time, he did not know that he would also find part of the answer to his asthma problems by finding the answers to my problems. As he began to research foods that could have a negative effect on triglycerides and cholesterol levels, he decided to look at what foods could have an adverse effect on asthma. What he found was that a lot of foods that we enjoyed eating were triggers for, not only allergic reactions, but also for asthma attacks. For example, he found that dairy products, such as milk and cheese could cause excess mucus production in some asthmatics. So he began to experiment with different recipes by removing dairy products to see if these changes reduced the chances of his suffering an asthma attack. If he had a chicken enchilada topped with cheese, he would have a mild asthma attack. If he used a dairy-based coffee creamer in his coffee, he would experience tightness in his chest and shortness of breath. He found that casein, the main protein found in milk and cheese products, increased his risk of developing a noticeable shortness of breath and in some cases would lead to asthma attacks of various degrees. So he decided to limit, and in some cases remove, milk and cheese products from his diet to see if there was any improvement in his daily asthma maintenance.

He replaced dairy creamers with coconut cream powder in his coffee. In his case, this has proved to be beneficial for two reasons. First, by eliminating cow's milk, he will avoid having an asthma attack. Second, after looking at the benefits of coconut milk, he found that some studies have shown that coconut milk and oil will induce satiety (the feeling of fullness) and decrease hunger. Almost immediately he noticed that he was eating smaller portions for lunch and dinner and that he was not getting hungry between meals. Because he was eating fewer calories, he was having more success in controlling his weight. Although he knew that coconut products were high in plant-based saturated fats and calories, he made it a point to use the coconut cream powder, sparingly.

In the spring of 2005, he also made a major discovery about what was also triggering his asthma and bringing on his attacks. While making raisin nut bread, he decided to add golden raisins, along with the regular raisins, to the recipe. Shortly after eating several slices of the bread, he began to experience shortness of breath and was in the beginning stages of a major asthma attack. After getting control of his breathing, he needed to find out why he had this attack. So he took an inventory of what he had eaten the entire day. He was perplexed because nothing appeared to be different. He began to look at the labels of everything he used to prepare the bread. Then he realized that we had never used golden raisins before this occasion. On the label was one thing that stood out—the preservative, sulfite. He immediately began researching the connection between sulfites and asthma. He found that this class of preservative, the sulfites, could trigger severe asthma attacks in some asthmatics. Sulfites can be found in numerous processed foods, including some dairy products. So this was also another consideration as to why some dairy products caused his difficulty in breathing.

Unfortunately, any type of sulfite preservative would later prove to be major triggers for his difficulty in breathing and, eventually, having an asthma attack. Shortly after the bread experience, he made a chili garlic sauce with our stir-fry for dinner. Later that evening, he began to experience a tightening in his chest. Although we had not eaten anything new, we took an inventory and tried to figure out what could have caused his reaction. Once again, we read the labels on all the foods that we had used to prepare our dinner. We found that a bi-sulfite preservative was used in this particular brand of hot garlic sauce. Although, in the past he found that the capsicum in hot peppers helped to break up the mucus and, in most cases, restored his normal breathing quickly, if the chili product contains sulfites, then the sulfites will be counterproductive in preventing and controlling his asthma attacks.

He did not think that part of the answer to his ongoing battle with asthma could be this easy. So he decided to experiment with this new knowledge. He took a teaspoon of chili garlic sauce without any preservatives and waited for a problem to arise. Fortunately, he did not experience any breathing problems. He then tempted fate by eating a small amount of the chili garlic sauce which contained sulfites and shortly afterwards began experiencing a slight tightening in his chest and a difficult breathing pattern. For him, any sulfite preservative appeared to be a major trigger for an asthma attack. His new plan of attack, no pun intended, was to ensure that any products we use do not contain any of the class of preservatives in the sulfite family.

This can, however, be problematic, because when eating out

it is not possible to know with exact certainty whether the food will contain a sulfite. For example, on our anniversary, we went to a Mexican restaurant. He ordered a meal that did not contain cheese and used no creamer for his coffee, but ate the tortilla chips with the salsa. Within a few hours, he began to experience a slight shortness of breath. We can only assume that the restaurant salsa, like many store brands often do, contained a sulfite preservative. This is something that we will continually learn to look for and try to avoid. If he is not sure, then he won't eat it. Another restaurant food which may contain a sulfite is any type of frozen potato. Many manufacturers are allowed to use sulfites to "preserve" the white color of the potato and the crunch. Without this preservative, pre-packaged potatoes would brown and become soggy after cooking. At restaurants, his only option is to ensure that only freshly cut potatoes are prepared on site. In his case, being able to breathe without any problems and avoid an asthma attack is worth giving up certain foods.

By eliminating foods with sulfites, he is able to breathe better. This has a spillover effect, in that he can now exercise more regularly because he feels healthier. Because of this, he is also able to take longer walks and hikes without experiencing breathing problems. At times, he would have to take shorter walks or hikes because his breathing was labored. Also, if it was a high ozone day, this would also make his breathing problematic. When asthmatics begin to have shortness of breath, they can get a little anxious which can prevent them from breathing properly, which in turn increases their shortness of breath and raises anxiety. This can be a vicious cycle that can have no end, especially if you are the one that cannot breathe. You may know that you need to control your anxiety to control your breathing, but if you cannot breathe it is hard to relax and do what is necessary to control the attack. It is scary to think that you may not be able to get to your medication or even a hospital in time because you could not make it back home because of an asthma attack. So, for him finding another trigger for his asthma and then being able to eliminate the trigger was a step in the right direction. This is about being proactive and finding solutions to control your problem.

Over the past three years, he has lost over 25 pounds and has not gained any of the weight back. As of the fall 2005, his cholesterol level and all his blood levels were normal. More importantly, he is feeling better than he has in years. During this past summer, while trying to perfect our camp-style of cooking with our new way of eating, he managed to break the 205-pound limit and went down to 200 pounds. He has been able to maintain this weight for the past few months and now has a new goal—190 pounds. With continual patience and healthy eating I know he will be able to meet this challenge.

In January 2008, the result of Kip's blood tests showed that his total cholesterol was 169, with this HDL and LDL cholesterol levels both within optimal ranges, and his triglyceride level was 96. Because his test results were all well within normal range, he was told that he would not need to get blood tests until his next annual exam. Although, I was extremely happy for him, I could not help but feel a twinge of jealousy. However, I recognized that many things in my personal life were not in balance, so I knew that I needed to work on getting things back in balance. This left me with the resolve to tighten up my rules of eating much better and adhering to stricter portion control; and to ensure I pay more attention to all the aspects of all my health and food choices.

The only thing Kip needs to continue to work on is his weight. When he changed jobs, the parking lot was located next to his building. He was no longer briskly walking 15-20 minutes daily, each way from his car to the building where his office was located and back to his car. And, with the longer commute leading to the lack of available exercise time, he gained some weight. And now that we are in Albuquerque, he still had a great parking space which prevents him from walking and getting more exercise. But, now he has more time to exercise on a daily basis. We still make time to take long walks and hike in the national park, on trails along the *bosque* (the "forest" area along the Rio Grande), and walk to the local dog park every day, weather permitting.

The specific things that Kip continues to look into and research are the possible food and environmental triggers regarding his asthma. For him, this is the one area that he will always have to pay extra attention to and make any necessary changes. As long as he is aware of what foods have the potential to aggravate his asthma and does what he needs to get his weight under control, the easier it will be for him to ensure that his diet remains healthy and promotes freer breathing.

A New Road on Our Journey

We have returned to our journey. We are in the process of beginning a new and different journey in a new city. We are still pleased with a "diet" that fits our lifestyle and what we wanted for ourselves. We have both found the things that we know we can control in our lives and we can be proactive about making the changes necessary to reach our goals. We continue to take natural and vitamin supplements. We continue to follow our personal dietary plan. Hopefully, with a new doctor I will continue to make progress toward controlling my triglyceride and cholesterol levels. I am optimistic that the changes I made worked for me and some of changes you decide to try may work for you, as well.

For me, the easiest thing is the dietary part of my lifestyle plan, because no one knows that I'm on a diet unless I take the time to explain why I eat what I eat. I have found that if one finds an easy and manageable way to prepare and enjoy foods, then one can find the way to healthier eating that is not unforgiving and punitive. Many diets that I tried forced me to cleanse or fast for periods of time, took away too many foods that I enjoyed, and did not consider my tradition or culture in setting dietary standards. This not only set me up for failure but it disrespected me as a person. So, in the end my husband and I gave up very few of the things we normally ate. We just learned how to prepare our favorite and traditional dishes differently.

For example, in his New Mexico Green Chili stew, we replaced the white potatoes with pinto beans. We will prepare chicken or vegetable fajitas, with corn or whole-wheat flour tortillas. Another example, every year, the first Saturday of November, my husband hosts a "Ghost Supper." This is part of his culture and traditional for his people and similar to *Dia de los Muertos*, "Day of the Dead" (November 2nd) which is tradition for the Mexican culture, my culture. For him, Ghost Supper celebrates the people in our lives that have passed on. We cook all day (without tasting the food as it is prepared). After he blesses the food at sunset, our guests eat and spend time with us, hoping some are "visited" by loved ones that have passed. For the supper, we still prepare roasted turkey with dressing, wild rice, corn soup, blackberry and pumpkin/sweet potato pies and fresh homemade "Indian bread," just to name a few of the dishes. In recent years, many of our guests have been surprised that what we serve is actually healthy and do not break any of our diet rules because of how we prepare the meal. However, sometimes, I still have to remind myself about portion control and eating in moderation because the food tastes so good.

In the end, my husband and I have found a way to honor and respect our traditions, cultures, and personal lifestyles and still maintain a healthy way of eating. I hope that what you get out of this book is a healthier, more enjoyable way of preparing and eating the foods that honors and respects your traditions, cultures, and the way you live.

2

The Seven Steps to Change

How Do I Begin My Personal Journey?

ltimately, this is a question that only you can answer. Because I have high lipids and cholesterol health issues and my husband has asthma and several food allergies, our health problems are unique to the food choices we make for ourselves. What you need to do is look at what health issues you and your family may or may not have. For example, you may be lactose-intolerant and may therefore have to avoid milk and dairy products or you may have celiac disease, in which case you cannot have products which contain gluten. As I said, your journey may also take into account any lifestyle choices you have consciously made, such as the decision to become a vegetarian or a vegan. Each person's journey must be respected and honored. Unfortunately, many of today's traditional "diets" tend to minimize the importance of our cultural, traditional and personal preferences we, as individuals, include in our dietary decisions.

Just as my husband and I addressed our likes and dislikes within each food group and blended these with our traditional and cultural dishes, you will need to do the same for yourself and your family. Because tastes and traditions are unique to each family and are always growing and changing, it is safe to assume that this process will always be ongoing for you, as well. And the types of processed foods made available to consumers are no exception, as more and more products are constantly being improved to meet the changing needs of the majority of consumers. This increases what foods you can adapt to your new diet. The more you look at the variety within each of the food groups, the more you will naturally change and expand your selections. Let's look at the steps that are necessary so that you can begin to make healthier changes in your diet and lifestyle.

First: When making any changes to your diet or lifestyle, you need to recognize that change is necessary and that you will be prepared to make a commitment toward change.

I call this a moment of "epiphany" or even "light-bulb" moment. If you do not believe that changes are necessary, then you will not be ready to make any changes and you will not be able to maintain changes that you make. So, you will need to take an honest look at what you feel you need to change. For myself, I knew I needed to lower my triglyceride and cholesterol levels, and maybe as a bonus lose a few pounds.

With my family history of adult onset Type 2 Diabetes, among other chronic illnesses, I knew that without controlling my diet and, in turn, my blood levels, I would eventually have a higher risk of developing Type 2 Diabetes, as well. In July 1993, my maternal grandmother died from complications of Type 2 Diabetes; all fourteen of my mother's siblings are Type 2 Diabetic; and five of them have high blood pressure. In October 2003, my maternal aunt passed away from a diabetes-related complication, after suffering a massive stroke. In January 2006, my mother also suffered a stroke, which was a direct result of her diabetes, and passed away. My older sister was diagnosed with Type 2 Diabetes before her 49th birthday. In August 2005, one maternal aunt and, in July 2007, one maternal uncle died of colon cancer. On my paternal side, one of my aunts and two of my uncle's are diabetic and my father had high blood pressure.

Although I knew that the odds were stacked against me, I believed that because I had always been on the thinner side, I would be immune to having any type of conditions that could be related to Type 2 Diabetes. As a young woman, I never did have the trouble controlling my weight, as my mother and older sister. I never had to go on "fad" diets to lose unwanted weight. I was always the "skinny" one in the family, along with my younger sister. I was not in complete denial about the family disease, but I never thought that I would have the problems of my grandmother, aunts and uncles, and mother before I was 50 or even 55 years old. I rationalized that once I began to have extreme problems with controlling my weight, only then would I run the risk of becoming an adult diabetic. So, even though I was slightly heavier than normal, I was still not overweight. I did not feel the need to do anything constructive about the slight weight gain.

It took a class project to motivate me into losing the "few pounds" that I had gained. It was not the prospect of becoming a diabetic or having any suspicion that I had a medical problem that could lead to diabetes. It was not until August 1999 that I came to the realization that I had a real medical condition. When I received the devastating news that my triglycerides level was over slightly over 1000, this was my "epiphany" or "light bulb" moment. At this point, I was forced to RECOGNIZE that change was necessary AND that I had to be PREPARED to make the commitment to change.

For some that have no immediate health concerns, it may be simply to lose a few pounds because you want to feel better and look better. For others, it may be to either prevent, delay, or control for a specific illness or disease. And still for others, that are comfortable with their current weight or have no immediate health concerns, you may simply want to eat healthier and engage in a healthier lifestyle.

For whatever reason you RECOGNIZE that change is necessary AND you may now be PREPARED to make the commitment to change, you need to understand what may be necessary to MAKE CHANGE. It is very easy for any diet/weight loss program to state that a person needs to make their changes for the better. However, what I found was that they did not give me the necessary tools I needed to understand how to implement changes into my own life on a permanent basis. It was easy for me to state that I needed to make permanent changes in my life, but I did not know how to start. At first, I was left with more questions than answers. How does one start? Where does one begin to look for these "changes" that they need to make? How does one know the difference?

For myself, I found myself at a loss for some answers. In one respect, I was luckier than most people. My husband was always proactive about his health and health-related issues. As a social worker, he was always interested in reading about new findings in medical health and mental health issues. He was able to guide me into how to become more proactive about my own health issues. He gave me basic advice on how to become more proactive and how to advocate for yourself, especially when talking to your healthcare provider. We talked about what I wanted to accomplish and what we, as a couple, would need to do in order to accomplish any goals we set for ourselves. These next two "steps" are something that we both came up with in order to help us make the necessary and permanent changes.

Second: You need to become health literate and proactive in the health decisions made between you and your doctor.

This is the step that my husband, as a social worker, believes is very important. If you do not invest in obtaining a certain amount of health literacy, then you are left at mercy of allowing your health providers to make all of your health decisions for you and family members. One needs to become aware of what and how illnesses and disease can affect you both on a short term basis and long term basis. If you have a medical moment of "epiphany," as I did in the fall of 1999, then this is the point that you need to begin to educate yourself about illness and disease. But, if you are lucky and do not have any urgent medical problems, and just want to improve your overall eating habits, you still should take the time to become health literate. You may be healthy now, but you may at some future point need to have some level of medical knowledge, either for yourself or even a family member. You need to become health literate. So, what does it mean to be health literate? According to Healthy People 2010, health literacy is:

"The degree to which individuals have the capacity to obtain, process, and understand basic health information and services needed to make appropriate health decisions."

While, health literacy includes the interaction between patients and their doctors, along with other professionals, also known as providers, in the healthcare system, this is not the only area of focus in becoming health literate. It is important that one become proactive in their medical/healthcare treatment options and plans. There a several ways in which one can measure whether or not a person is health literate. But health literacy needs to come, not only from the patient to the health providers, but also from the health providers to the patient.

First, a patient who is health literate is comfortable in asking questions regarding health issues from their provider because their healthcare provider has the ability to listen. Second, the patient needs to understand what is needed to improve their health because their provider takes the time to clearly describe the treatment options and plans. Third, the patient has access to healthcare services because their provider advises on the best ways to enter the necessary system of care. Lastly, a patient engages in appropriate decision making regarding their healthcare options because their provider advised them with all of the necessary information regarding treatment options and plans.

In return, healthcare provider must be open to their patients' background. While certain illnesses and diseases need to be treated in similar manners, the healthcare provider needs to recognize that every patient is different. In order for this to occur, one needs to endure that their provider tries to become as culturally competent a provider as possible. First, the healthcare provider needs to have a certain level of cultural awareness so that the patient feels that they are respected. Second, the provider needs to show linguistic competence so that their patient is fully able to understand their directions and is able to process both verbal and non-verbal health-related information. Third, the provider needs to use cultural appropriateness so that the treatment plans can take into account the cultural attitudes of the patient. Lastly, the provider needs to show cultural sensitivity so that the healthcare information they are trying to send to their patient can reflect the patients' values.

As I stated, my mother was not health literate. And as I would soon find out, her doctors were not culturally competent providers. This situation between her and her providers lead to her becoming even less health literate and would lead to a host of healthcare misinformation and misunderstandings. Whenever she went to the doctor she would just listen to him tell her what the results of her blood glucose tests and briefly discuss her diet and exercise routines. I remember asking her how she was doing; she would get this sad look on her face and she would reply "fine." I knew by her tone in her voice that something was wrong. One day, she asked if I would go with her to her doctor's appointment. Of course, I agreed. But, I asked her why she wanted me there with her. She said that her regular doctor was on vacation and that another member of the doctors group would be seeing her. She stated she was afraid of him because he always "yelled" at her for not "controlling her sugar." When we arrived, this one doctor seemed a bit gruff and to the point, but did not appear to be "yelling" at her.

What I saw as one of the problems was that my mother always viewed her doctors as authority figures. They were highly educated, and therefore, never wrong and should never be questioned. When she went to the doctors, she would simply sit there quietly and listen to what was said, not fully understanding what was being explained. She would be asked if she understood, but was too afraid to tell the doctors that she did not understand exactly what they were telling her about her diabetes. When I went with her, this one doctor looked directly at her, exhaled in a somewhat bothersome tone, and simply said, "Mrs. Medina, you are not controlling your sugar. Your A1C is too high. It is 10.5." Then he said he was going to increase her medication for three months to see if this would lower this level and ordered another blood glucose test, as well. Lastly, he stated that if he was not happy with her progress, she would "be forced to go on insulin injections."

When I asked him what the A1C level meant, he did not take the time to explain, but simply directed me to his physicians' assistant (PA). When I asked the PA what the results of the A1C blood test meant, she stated, and I quote, "I don't know. Diabetics just need to have this level routinely tested." These answers and treatment by her healthcare providers left my mother near tears and in a more stressful condition than when she first arrived at the office. Needless to say, I left the office very upset and angry. I could see why my mother was afraid of her doctors and not health literate. Her doctor, an older Anglo male, did not fully understand my mother's culture and her issues with those in authority, while my mother was too timid to question her doctors or her test results. Although, she knew her fasting blood glucose was always within range, she did not understand what the A1C level meant. She did not know how to approach the doctor to ask the proper questions. For example, she never asked the obvious question. Why, if her fasting blood glucose is always within normal range, is her A1C always showing that she is "not controlling her sugar?" They both played into each others' failure to properly communicate with each other. So I had to become more health literate regarding Type 2 Diabetes in order to assist my mother. In the process, I also became my mother's health advocate.

The first thing I did was to go to the local bookstore and pick up a medical reference book on medical tests. I found out what the A1C test was and why it was important in showing a doctor whether or not a diabetic is controlling their "sugar." I also looked up all the other blood glucose-related tests. I had to educate myself so that her doctor would be answering my questions. During her next visit, as he went over her improved results, I intervened by asking for specific answers to the medical information he asked her. I also intervened by answering his questions to her about her diet and exercise plans. In some way, I forced him to take the time to really hear my mother's concerns and my mother became more empowered to see that there were some questions he could not answer. The doctor also became aware that my mother was no longer going to be a passive patient, and was willing to become more proactive in her healthcare treatment. While, my mother was never fully health literate, she at least became more knowledgeable about some of the basic information she needed to make better decisions about her health. In the end, she formed a better relationship with her doctor, not perfect, but one in which he took the time to talk TO her and not AT her. Ultimately, what I found out about "routine" blood glucose tests has helped me to understand my own health problems. I am a very proactive health literate patient.

Basically, in order to become health literate, you need to take the time to understand what the results of certain "routine" tests actually mean. It is not enough for a patient to depend on the healthcare provider to tell you what the results mean. These are your test results, your health, and in the end your healthcare decisions. You need to become knowledgeable because the more you understand, the better you will be able to follow your healthcare plan that you and your provider develop. I routinely look up the standard acceptable blood glucose levels, so that I always know, before I go in for my doctor's appointment, whether or not the standards have changed. Also, I want to know whether or not my levels are within the normal, borderline, or high range.

If specialized or additional tests are ordered, you should be confident to ask the provider why the test or tests are being ordered. You, as the patient, have the right to know why tests are being ordered and what medical issues the provider is looking for or what medical issues the provider is ruling out. This gives you the opportunity to look into what the provider may be looking for as a diagnosis. For example, when I told my provider that my maternal aunt was diagnosed with end stage colon cancer, he ordered a colonoscopy. Although, I was only 49 years old at the time, my doctor stated that because I have colon cancer in my family, this raises my risk for developing this often fatal disease. When caught early, colon cancer can often be treated. This test is usually done at age 50, then every five years so long as the test is negative. Because I now had family history, one year before most people get their first colonoscopy, this test was ordered for me. Days before my colonoscopy, I began an internet search, using several reliable medical websites, and read everything I could find out about colonoscopy, the test results, and colon cancer treatment. I was fully prepared before the date of my test to ask the appropriate questions that I may have needed to ask. I did not wait until after I got the results. I wanted to be fully prepared at the time of the test. This is something that a proactive health literate patient would do.

In the April 2008 edition of *Diabetes Forecast*, there was an article entitled, "Get In The Game," which gave information on the importance of building a diabetes health care team. After reading this article, I found that the basic information can actually apply to any major illness or disease. This article reported that your point person, in your inner circle of healthcare needs, should be your family practice or primary care physician (PCP), along with their physician's assistant or nurse practitioner. Usually for a person with diabetes this would be an endocrinologist. Your PCP is instrumental is getting you the proper referrals for any specialists you may need to consult. Therefore, according to the article, it is imperative that you form a positive relationship with your physician. Others that need to be in your inner circle include a nurse educator, registered dietician, eye doctors, such as an optometrist and/or ophthalmologist, and a dentist.

According to this article, as your healthcare needs change, you may need to add other specialists, as the "second string" of your healthcare team, which include mental health professionals, pharmacists, foot doctor or podiatrist, and other healthcare specialists. For example, this article states that a diabetic may need to be referred to a nephrologist or a kidney doctor, a person with heart trouble may need to be referred to a cardiologist or heart doctor, and those needing surgery may need a referral to a surgical specialist. It is a matter of you understanding why each of these specialist are being referred to you and what the specialist is expected to treat and the prognosis. No matter what, this article also states what I have come to understand and believe—there is no "I" in T-E-A-M. You, the patient, are the most important decision-maker—the "captain"—of the team. Therefore, you need to track your test results, take your medication, eat healthy foods, and exercise regularly; so that you will be able to recognize any problems or changes.

Third: You need to recognize the difference between diet/weight loss plans and healthy eating.

This step became necessary because I found there is a lot of misinformation about diets and dietary programs. What I did know about diet/weight loss plans was that they did not work for me, as I struggled to lose weight and lower my triglyceride and cholesterol levels. I tried to figure out why I kept failing. Using the "health literacy" approach, I began to research diet/weight loss programs the same way I would any specific illness or disease, such as my mother's Type 2 Diabetes or my diagnosis of Hyperlipidemia or high triglycerides and Hypercholesterolemia or high cholesterol. I began to research foods and food groups and how they interacted with the body. Although, my husband already had a substantial amount of knowledge about foods, he allowed me to research and find things out for myself. What I eventually found out was not that surprising to me in some respects, while totally surprising in others.

Simply stated, for many people trying to lose weight, some dieting/weight loss plans turn out to be a temporary phase and a quick fix. So, in some cases, the weight loss is temporary, then for some reason - usually you've lost all the weight you can at the time - you hit the plateau and cannot lose the rest of the weight you want. At this point, you will give up and try another plan to lose more weight or you will give up and gain the weight back. Sometimes you may even gain more weight than you originally lost. Unfortunately, some of these diet plans do not give you the tools you need to make the changes permanent. I believe this is because most of these dieting/weight loss plans, however well intentioned, do not consider your needs as an individual or your family and friends as a part of your world. More importantly, they do not consider or recognize the connection and interaction between you and your extended family and friends as an instrumental part of the process of the healthy eating process.

This "step" is something that I felt was necessary because of how I was educated about diets, in general. I learned all of my dieting/weight loss "tricks" and secrets from my mother. In 1967, we moved to the west side of Chicago. Although my mother was happy about our new house, she was not an emotionally happy person. A few years earlier she lost her father and she went into an emotional tailspin. She found that by eating "comfort" foods she felt better, but this lead to her gaining an enormous amount of weight. She went from approximately 120 pounds to approximately 220—225 pounds. At approximately 5' 1", she was not just obese, but morbidly obese. About three years later, she heard about a new weight loss program that promoted weekly meetings, along with group support, she decided to join. She convinced three other neighbors that had similar weight issues to join the local area church-sponsored Weights Watchers Program with her. Together, the four women lost a combined weight of 350 pounds in a two year period. My mother reached her goal weight of 135 pounds, just in time for my elementary school graduation.

Just as she and her fellow members were managing their weight, several things happened to stop their progress. First, the church stopped sponsoring the program. Then several of the group members moved away to neighborhoods too far away to keep their group together. This left my mother with very little support. She and the remaining two began to regain the weight they initially lost. At first, it was very little; a few pounds here, a few pounds there.

Then they would begin a yo-yo period of weight loss and weight gain. Over time, without the support of all the group members and the program, all four regained the weight they lost while on the program. A few, including my mother, gained more weight than they originally lost.

This was when my mother began to try any "fad" diet that she heard of or read about. She tried various diets she read about in magazines, including the grapefruit or "Hollywood" diet, the mineral water diet, the cabbage soup diet, and numerous fasting diets which required her to basically starve herself for short periods. Although many of these worked for a while and she would lose weight, she could not stay on any of them long enough to make a lasting difference. This yo-yo weight period in her life lasted about 18 years. It was not until May 1985, when weighing approximately 235 pounds, she was diagnosed a Type 2 Diabetic. At this point, my mother knew she had to find some way to lose the weight and keep it off. This was her moment of "epiphany" and she recognized that change was needed and that she was ready to make the changes.

The one thing that really allowed her to get control of her weight was the fact that her doctor was also a diagnosed Type 2 Diabetic. He was able to relate and empathize with what she would be going through. He was also able to talk to her, as one diabetic to another, and give her some helpful suggestions about what she needed to eat. Although, she lost the weight, she was never able to fully understand why or how certain foods she continued to eat still could create future problems with her blood glucose levels. She just relied on his "expertise" to know what she needed to do and to tell her what she needed to do. And she would transfer this way of thinking onto all of her future doctors. Her doctors would always know what was in her best interest.

When I was "dieting," my family and friends would unknowingly sabotage my attempts to eat healthier. When I eliminated my "comfort" foods and the foods that I enjoyed which were not allowed as part of my new "diet," I did not need anyone to help sabotage my diet plans. If I was invited to their home for dinner or to a restaurant, there were usually lots of foods available that I was not allowed to eat or had eliminated from my "diet." To avoid hurt feelings and making others uncomfortable with my individual and restrictive diet requirements, I would make the choice to temporarily go off my diet.

Healthy eating should be about making a permanent change in your eating habits for the overall health of you and your family and not just focused on the one issue of weight loss. In a healthy eating plan, you need to explore what you do that is healthy then focus and expand on this. Do not get bogged down on what you think you are doing wrong or unhealthy in your current eating habits. If you find something that is not a healthy choice, you can correct it by either eliminating it or by working to make it a healthier choice. In most cases, you will only need to eliminate some of the more highly processed foods, which in most cases contain unhealthy additives.

Being a native Chicagoan, I have always loved pizza and did not want to eliminate it. But I needed to find a way I could keep pizza a part of healthy eating. While on a visit to Chicago a few years back, I found a pizzeria that made an excellent broccoli pizza. This made me look at what I specifically liked about pizza. I started to experiment with different toppings, while my husband worked on perfecting a homemade whole wheat pizza crust and pizza sauce. We top our pizza with a variety of vegetables and will sometimes add turkey pepperoni. However, we go very light on the cheese to make a true Italian-style pizza. Because cheese is one of his asthma triggers, my husband eats his pizza without the cheese, instead using olive oil drizzled lightly on top. So with very few changes, we were both able to keep pizza a part of our healthy eating plan. I have realized that although my journey for healthy eating is a permanent change in my life and in my family's life, there will always be room to make changes necessary to adapt and incorporate different foods.

Also, because of my family traditions in a Mexican-American family, I was brought up eating foods that directly reflected my culture. One of the earliest memories I remember is that of helping my mother prepare homemade white flour tortillas for us. She would wrap a large dish towel around my waist and stand me on a chair against the stove with a spatula. She would roll out the tortillas one by one and place them on the hot *comal* (flat pan) to cook. It was my job to turn them over and then carefully place them in the container. She would make three to four dozen at least twice a week, and sometimes as many as three times a week. My father would always expect the homemade tortillas and this became a staple of our family diet and incorporated into every meal. I remember that on the weekends, after having bacon and eggs, my mother would save the bacon grease and use it in her tortillas, if we could not afford to buy lard or shortening. Then when she would make *frijoles de olla*, she would refry the beans in either the bacon grease or oil. Whenever she made Spanish rice, she would add a little oil to brown the white rice before she added the tomatoes, spices and water before she brought the rice to simmer. Without realizing it, I grew up with a lot of saturated fats and white food products in my diet. These foods and this way of cooking became my ultimate "comfort" foods because they represented all that made me feel good and safe. It was easy to mimic the way my mother cooked, because she in fact taught me all of her cooking secrets.

> **Fourth:** You need to take an inventory of what you and your family eats.

This is the easiest way to see if you and your family have poor diet control. Not eating a proper well-balanced diet can create an increased potential for a variety of health-related problems. Taking an inventory helps you to recognize how much you may be overindulging and overeating certain foods, in general. You need to take a close look at what your daily caloric intake is and how much you are actually consuming. To do this you will need to start by keeping a daily food journal. This can be the hardest thing to do because it requires taking an honest look at how much you actually consume. Many people can be in denial about how much they actually eat. On the positive side, this helps you to recognize what foods are traditions for your family, as well as, what foods are personal preferences. This helps you to evaluate typical meals and understand how the "extras," such as desserts and snacks, are part of your daily diet.

For a woman my height, I should have been eating approximately 1,500 to 1,700 calories daily. After I charted my eating habits for a few days, I realized I was in denial about how much I was actually consuming on a daily basis. I made simple mistakes. I did not realize that my average serving sizes were much larger than they were supposed to be. I was shocked to see that I ate between 2,000 and 2,300 calories a day. Not only was I eating an extra meal, but the foods were higher in "hidden" sugars, higher in "hidden" and "wrong" fats, higher in "wrong" carbohydrates, higher in calories, and lower in fiber. Also, I would eat without realizing. I was eating because the food was available and I had the opportunity to eat. I found it was especially easy to snack endlessly while watching television. This is why a book that lists the fat, carbohydrate, and calorie content was important. It gave me the perspective I needed to be honest about how much I was actually eating.

I recommend purchasing a book that lists the calorie, fat, carbohydrate, and fiber content of foods. The book that I found to be useful for myself was *The Doctor's Pocket Calorie, Fat & Carbohydrate Counter* by Allen Borushek, Dietician and "Calorie King." When preparing meals at home, it gave me a basic understanding of how many calories, fats, and carbohydrates are in specific foods and what the average serving sizes should be. When my husband and I travel, we cannot cook our own meals and, therefore, we are at a disadvantage. We are left with no choice but to eat out at restaurants. This particular book lists 170 fast food chains and restaurants. We are able to look up menus and make healthy decisions on not only where to stop and eat, but what to choose ahead of time. So when we order, it is not obvious that we are "dieting." If a specific restaurant is not listed in the book, we try to match it as closely as possible to one that is and make an appropriate selection. This helped us learn about portion control, as well. In general, I consider this type of book an excellent guide for those who want to begin to monitor and change their eating habits.

This step turned out to be a good step in the right direction. According to an April 2008 *Time Magazine* article, entitled "Dear (Food) Diary," it was reported that a new study found that those dieters who kept a food diary doubled their weight loss, when compared to the non-diary dieters. Nearly 1,700 overweight or obese adults at least 25 years old were tracked for the study. All of the participants were encouraged to use and given weight-loss maintenance strategies, such as calorie restrictions, weekly group sessions, moderately intensive exercise, and keeping a food journal. Six months later, researchers reported that of those in the study, participants who used a food journal lost an average of 18 pounds compared to an average of 9 pounds of the non-diary participants. Researchers believe that it was not just the recording of the foods consumed that led to the higher weight loss. The researchers stated that by recording what you eat, the person becomes aware of their eating habits and can readily identify eating habits that need to be modified. Lastly, the researchers reported that while many people believe they can remember what they eat, many tend to only have a general idea as to what they eat and how much they actually consume. Many people in the study were able to see exactly where the extra calories came from.

Fifth: You need to take an inventory of what is in your cupboard and pantry.

This is the natural next step when taking a personal inventory of what you and your family eats. Just as in the second step, this step allows you to become healthier food and healthy food literate. This step allows you to take better control of what you eat, what your family eats, and how you prepare the foods you purchase for consumption. When understanding why certain foods are instrumental to good health and why certain foods are detrimental to long term health, you become food literate. Many people simply want to make a purchase and not have to think about what is in the product or how the product is made. Consumers like the ease of going into a grocery store and buying what they want from an unlimited selection.

It is imperative that one understand the relationship between foods, especially highly processed foods, and your body, so you can then make better choices, healthier choices. In order to rid your body of the "bad" hidden foods you must also rid your cupboard and pantry of these things, as well. Simply stated, if these foods are not in your house, you will be less likely to consume them. Once you begin purchasing the healthier foods that you and your family enjoy eating, you can begin a healthier way of eating and start your personal journey to health and wellness. You can start by simply following my four basic rules of eating and four basic rules of shopping (see Chapter Three).

During this step, I became a more informed consumer and realized the shopping mistakes I made were easy to correct. I freely admit I was an uninformed, naive consumer. I used to purchase whichever ready-made processed pasta sauce, baked beans, bread, peanut butter, etc. that I liked and, as a bonus, saved money because these products were on sale or I had a coupon to redeem. In this step, by reading the labels on all the products, I found that almost everything I purchased contained unhealthy hidden additives. I did not realize the amount of added processed sugars, "bad" fats, and actual calories I was eating.

Also, as consumers become more health conscious, products available at the markets will change based on what consumers want. Two of the more popular diet plans, such as Atkins and South Beach, which have their own brand name products, have forced many manufacturers to "take inventory of their own cupboards and pantries." Some manufacturers have released "new," "improved," and "healthy" products to keep up with the consumers' demand for these types of healthier foods. Currently, there is a trend to change the makeup of processed foods, such as breads, cereals, and snack products. More of these products are being made with whole grains and multi grains and have no trans fats. Also other products, such as margarines, are being made without trans fats and have added heart-healthy cholesterol-lowering ingredients. Now, yogurts are getting a healthy makeover, as well. There is an extended choice of yogurts that are fortified with, not only cholesterol-lowering ingredients, but with probiotics—healthy bacteria. These probiotics place healthy bacteria in your intestinal tract; helping to regulate your digestive system and assisting the body in removing unhealthy or "bad" bacteria.

Sixth: If you remove something, you should add or replace it with something else.

My husband and I found this step was crucial to combining our new healthier dietary plan with our combined traditions. We used this very simple and basic behavioral modification technique. When I took my psychology course in behavior modification, I thought I understood the importance of removing and eliminating unhealthy foods. While my mind understood this, my body did not understand this and would still crave what was "normal" food. Because I was not getting an enjoyable immediate replacement or any type of immediate reward in return, I began to resent the approach of many diet plans and diet programs. This is exactly why these types of diet plans failed for me. Changing to a healthier eating style should never be a negative experience or about punishing yourself and your family. Ultimately you will get to the point where you become frustrated and you will most likely fail and go back to the unhealthy way of eating.

Therefore, taking an immediate "replacement" approach helped me to become a more knowledgeable and proactive consumer and to learn more about basic nutrition. I decided that my only alternative was to try to remove the processed foods that specifically contained any unhealthy additives and replace them with better healthy choices, without compromising my basic dietary preferences. After researching specific foods and looking at the different food groups, I found that I already enjoyed eating foods that were beneficial for my health. For example, I like most vegetables, so eating some typical mixes and types, such as the California blend of broccoli, cauliflower, and carrots, were easy. To then make the leap and add other mixes and types of vegetables became easier. I started to limit the amount of rice, potatoes, and breads and eat more vegetables and vegetable mixes. Also, some tips are obvious, such as to replace whole milk with skim, 1%, or 2% milk, replace regular ice cream with fat-free sugar-free frozen yogurt or plain nonfat yogurt with fresh fruit, replace a chocolate shake with a blueberry smoothie, replace white bread with 100% whole-wheat or 100% whole grain breads, replace white rice with brown rice or wild rice, replace an occasional regular candy bar with sugar-free dark chocolate or occasional dark chocolate covered strawberries, limit or replace red meats with poultry and fish.

Seventh: You need to develop your own healthy diet according to your culture, tradition, and personal lifestyle preferences.

This final step may seem the most difficult, but it is actually the easiest one to incorporate and one that becomes an ongoing process. This is the point where you start your individualized "replacement" approach. Through incorporating those healthy foods that your family already enjoys eating with the foods that you like, but may need some modification, you will be able to tailor your own healthier way of eating. By doing this I was able to create a healthier way of eating, which includes many of my favorite Mexican and New Mexican dishes and other recipes that are an important part of my family history and tradition. In the end, I feel as if I am actually giving up very little of what my family members and I enjoy eating. Enjoying the foods you and your family eats are an integral part in maintaining your commitment to your new healthier eating plan.

By making an easy substitution of pinto beans for white potatoes in my green chili stew recipe, made the stew healthier and kept it in our diet. I still enjoy eating most of my favorite foods, such as tacos, fajitas, enchiladas, Mexican-style rice, pinto beans, corn bread, fry bread, corn soup, cream soups, stir-fry, gumbo, pies, and pancakes. The list of what I feel I didn't give up is almost endless. And more importantly, the list of foods I can use as replacements in recipes is just as endless. My husband's and my creativity in preparing the foods we eat is what helps to create a satisfying and healthy diet. And your creativity in the kitchen is what will make this way of eating satisfying for you and your family, as well. You just need to start buying, preparing, and enjoying the new, improved, and healthier foods of your family's new eating style. You will then be well on your way to your personal journey to health and healing.

3

Healthy Eating Basics

What to Eat, What Not to Eat, and How to Choose

What I found to be most discouraging throughout my experience in trying to find the best way to incorporate a healthy diet into my lifestyle was that I almost always went through periods of depression because of the restrictions that are required as part of the majority of diet programs. What I wanted to do was to just wake up one morning and start cooking and eating healthier without having to deny or deprive myself of foods that I was accustomed to eating. If I wanted to have pancakes and eggs for breakfast, tacos for lunch, pizza for dinner, and maybe dessert, I wanted to be able to do these things.

The trick with my way of eating is simple. I take what I like and in the case of unhealthy dishes I just prepare and cook them differently. However, there are changes you will have to make. The changes you need to make are removing or limiting the unhealthy choices in your current diet and replacing them with healthier choices. With your creative choices in the kitchen and in restaurants, you and your family can still eat "normal." Other diets make you fast or cleanse for weeks and deprive you of entire food groups, wean you back onto what food groups are allowed, or make you buy into food plans that offer prepared foods in pre-packaged serving sizes. These types of diets do not teach you how to maintain the plan after you no longer buy into them. Besides, one is faced with the reality of having to try and replicate these pre-packaged meals not only for yourself, but for your family, as well. This forces you to then prepare one meal for yourself and different meals for your family. Your kitchen becomes a restaurant and you become a short-order cook.

While doing the research on my medical conditions, I found that in order to maintain optimal reductions of triglycerides and cholesterol levels certain foods were recommended as part of a diet, exercise programs were encouraged, and various herbal and vitamin supplements were advised. These are standard recommendations for any diet/weight loss plan. I also found that many of the dietary recommendations on Internet medical sites and even some weight loss diet programs were very similar and in some cases identical. What I tried to do was to simply mesh similar advice on what types of foods to eat and what types of foods not to eat. This is where my personal dietary plan started to take shape. I knew I would have to try to come up with basic easy-to-follow rules, especially for my mother. Unfortunately this turned into a nightmare, because I wanted to include everything to stay on a healthy dietary plan. The more I read, the more I realized that my attempts to eat a healthier diet had turned into a complex monster of rules. At one point, I had about a dozen little rules to follow, with about four other rules attached to the original twelve.

So I decided to come up with fewer easier rules, which allowed me to alter the rest of my diet while still honoring my tradition, culture, and lifestyle. These basic rules are good for all people and everything else can be changed according to your traditions, culture, and personal health concerns. I found that by following these rules everything else fell into place and I no longer had to try to figure out what to do and how to do it. I learned how to be a more creative cook and I learned how to "eat better." Cooking is now a natural task and I do not starve until the next meal. I began by integrating the following four basic rules into my daily eating habits.

The Four Rules of Eating

1. "White" Is Bad

What I am specifically referring to are "White" flour products, "White" potatoes, and "White" rice. I also include refined sugars, which are high glycemic carbohydrates.

There are two type of carbohydrates; simple and complex. Simple carbohydrates, also known as simple sugars, include regular table sugar, fruit sugar, and milk sugar, as well as other types of sugars. On the other hand, complex carbohydrates, are also made up of sugars, but their sugar molecules are strung together to form much longer complex chains. Also, foods in the complex carbohydrate category also are made up of fiber and starches, which include whole grains, fruits and vegetables, and peas and beans. Both simple and complex carbohydrates are converted into glucose.

Generally speaking simple carbohydrates will metabolize in your system faster and can cause your blood glucose levels to spike rapidly. In sensitive individuals, simple carbohydrates can and will increase triglycerides and cholesterol levels. Obviously, this was one of my major problem areas, as I was a serious bread/tortilla/rice addict. Also, simple carbohydrates have a tendency to fill you up fast, but leave you feeling hungry earlier after eating. You learn that one serving is not enough. And the cycle of eating larger portions begins. I had to learn the importance of recognizing my limit and portion control.

A very important form of a carbohydrate is fiber, which in the past was also known as "bulk" or "roughage." Fiber is broken down into seven classifications; bran, cellulose, gum, hemicellulose, lignin, mucilages, and pectin. Each of these classifications has its own function. However, it is important to note that fiber is also broken down into two categories; soluble and insoluble. Soluble fiber dissolves in water and takes the form of a gel-like substance, which helps to soften the stools. Higher amounts of soluble fiber can be found in oats, legumes, apples, bananas, berries, barley, and some vegetables. Insoluble fiber is not dissolved in water and passes through the intestine and adds bulk to the stools. Higher amounts of insoluble fiber can be found in whole wheat and whole grain foods, bran, nuts, seeds, and the skin of some fruits and vegetables.

Fiber is necessary for many reasons; it helps the body to retain water and helps to bind with other substances that would normally result in the production of cholesterol, which then allows for the elimination of these substances from the body. Although, there are other terms used in discussing fiber, such as dietary fiber, functional fiber, and total fiber, it does not matter what form you are consuming. The thing that matters the most is the amount of total fiber you consume. Because fiber is important to healthy body function, on average, 60% of your total daily caloric intake should be in complex carbohydrates. Lastly, foods which are higher in fiber increase the feeling of satiety, the feeling of being full, than refined low-fiber foods. And whole foods high in fiber will also be lower in fat and calories, which are both helpful to lower cholesterol levels, lower blood glucose levels, and lower insulin levels. Therefore, in looking for a great tool to any weight loss or weight maintenance program, the key is to increase the amount of fiber you consume.

Whole grains are a good source of vitamin E and folate. Whenever purchasing whole-wheat and whole grain products, read the label very carefully. Sometimes just stating that the products are "whole" wheat and "whole" grain does not mean that they are 100% whole-wheat or 100% whole grain. In looking at Step Six, immediate replacement of foods, I found that instead of eating "White" breads, I replaced them with whole wheat and whole grains. Instead of prepared "White" flour pancake mixes, I would make my own whole grain flour pancakes. Instead of eating "White" rice, I replaced with brown and wild rice and other whole grains, such as quinoa. Also, there are many gluten-free alternatives in eating more whole grains for those who have other health issues, such as Celiac disease. For example, teff is rapidly growing in popularity. Teff, a whole grain from Africa, is one of the most nutrient-dense grains. Because of its small size, it is almost entirely made up of bran and endosperm, the most nutritious part of any grain. This particular grain is very versatile and can be used as a side, along any meat, poultry, or fish, or as a hot cereal and may be added to soups and stews. Another seed that is quickly gaining popularity is the Chia seed, which is better known by the general public as the novelty gift, the Chia pet, which grows its own "hair." This seed which is edible, is higher in Omega-3 fatty acids than flaxseed and, unlike flaxseeds, can be stored for long periods of time without going rancid and do not require grinding for consumption.

The key in adding whole grains is to try to be open to new types of grains, in order to broaden what you prepare for you and your family. Because I am a self-admitted "carbohydrate" addict, only eating whole grains did not make me feel deprived of a food group that I love. I have easily incorporated whole-wheat sugar-free breads, whole-wheat flour or corn tortillas, whole-wheat pastas, brown or wild rice, oats, oat bran, and rice bran into my dietary plan. To be honest I now like the taste of whole grains better, over plain and tasteless "white" breads. Although, baking with whole-wheat can be tricky, you need to be patient with whole grain flours.

Although, whole grain products are an excellent way to incorporate healthier carbohydrates into your eating plan, they are not the only complex carbohydrate. Just as one would replace "white" flour products and "white" rice with other whole grains, this is the same process you need to take with "white" potatoes. While potatoes do have some health benefits, this vegetable can have it drawbacks for those who are trying to control their "sugar." Many times it is what is added to the potato that makes it a bad dietary choice. For example, in a baked potato, one forgets the additional fats and calories come from the butter, sour cream, cheese, and bacon bits. Then add the protein and saturated fat, especially if it is red meat, portion of the meal. All of these additions, to an otherwise fairly good choice, make the potato a worse choice than simply adding a second vegetable or eating a smaller portion of meat. When preparing any variety of potato, I will always include the skin, which contains fiber.

Also, this is the point where I expanded my consumption of a wider variety of vegetables into my eating habits. Instead of opting for the usual potato side, I either added a second, higher fiber, nutrient-dense vegetable or just served a double helping of whatever vegetable I prepared. Although, I always liked the more typical vegetables, such as corn, peas, and green beans, there were a number of vegetables that I would simply not eat, ever. Because I was able to look at non-traditional vegetables from a different perspective, I found that I was able to, at the very least, give them a try. I was never a spinach eater, but now use it as a base for any salad; I use kale or Swiss chard in my curry sauce when making a veggie or chicken curry; and I replace a plain potato at every holiday meal with yams, sweet potatoes, or an acorn or butternut squash. I have even made *caldo*, Mexican beef stew, with chunks of turnips and rutabagas, in place of the standard white potato.

When I look at sugar, from a simple carbohydrate perspective, I use a slightly different approach. For me, the only sugar I felt I needed was in my coffee. I was never that into eating sweets, such as cakes, cookies, and candy. Sure, there were certain processed desserts I liked, but none that I loved to the point I could not give them up. Okay, maybe the Almond Joy and Mounds bars were difficult to stop eating, but I was able to break my "addiction" to them. Once I gave up the sugar in my coffee, I recognized the amount of sugar that was in other products. I remember going to a friend's house for his birthday. After the cake was cut, I accepted a very small piece in order to not upset the hostess. As I began to eat the cake, I could literally feel the sugar granules on my teeth; I could feel the fat, from the butter cream icing, along my lips and tongue. I felt as if I were eating a stick of butter that was rolled over table sugar. As I tried to eat this small piece, I tried to imagine how I ever thought this way of eating was pleasurable. Now, whenever I want something sweet, I go for something that is in its natural whole state. I will eat blueberries, cherries, apples, or any other fresh whole fruit for dessert. Whenever, I go to a buffet-style event, I always look for the fresh fruits and vegetables.

You often cannot easily eliminate all refined carbohydrates from your diet. I recognized that some of these carbohydrates were ingrained into my styles of eating. These were evident in almost all of my dietary choices; from choosing breads and tortillas, to choosing pasta and rice, and even to choosing certain vegetables. This was also evident in how I prepared my foods. I knew that I would not be able to give up all of them and go whole grain entirely. For example, I have always and will always like all types of rice, especially white rice. On occasion, I will still eat white jasmine rice, but I do so in moderation and I always add stabilized rice bran when preparing any type of white rice. Sometimes I will mix white jasmine rice with brown rice and/or wild rice. I recently found one particular brand which sells whole brown jasmine rice. Basically, I just try to always make the "100% whole grain" choices first.

2. No to "OSE"

This sounds silly. After all, what is an "OSE?" And, exactly where in any grocery store is the "OSE" aisle? What I am referring to is Sucrose and High Fructose Corn Syrup (HFCS).

Sucrose is the chemical name for regular white table sugar that has been refined from cane or beet juice. This process strips away all of its nutrients. Sucrose is a type of carbohydrate, but supplies "empty" calories to the body. As it metabolizes, sucrose breaks down in the intestine as glucose and fructose. HFCS, which is made from cornstarch, contains the two basic sugar building blocks, glucose and fructose, although not in equal proportion. HFCS is 45% glucose and 55% fructose. Therefore, fructose is absorbed into the body differently than glucose. Glucose releases leptin, which signals to your body that you are full so you eat less, and prevents the release of ghrelin, which makes you feel hungry. Fructose prevents fat cells from releasing leptin and does not suppress ghrelin. Fructose can increase hunger, thereby making you eat more. Also, the liver converts fructose into the chemical backbone of triglycerides more efficiently than is the case for glucose.

While several studies, including one by the University of California at Davis, show there is a clear difference in how fructose and glucose are metabolized in your body, these same studies do not show that fructose is worse than any other added sugar for your body. Many industries use this rationale to promote and validate the use of HFCS, as an additive, in many of their products. But, if you look at the statement for what it actually states and not how the statement is being manipulated to fit what the industry wants it to say, you will come to the basic conclusion that all added processed sugars in any form are equally as bad. In another study conducted by the University of Cincinnati Obesity Research Center (UCORC), which included overweight and/or obese men and women whose average age was 50 years, looked at the difference in type of added body fat by consuming fructose or glucose. During the trial, the study participants drank fructose- or glucose-sweetened beverages, totaling 25% of their daily caloric intake. The results of this study showed that both groups experienced added fat, however, for those in the fructose group added fat occurred in the belly, while those in the glucose group added fat under the skin or subcutaneous. Many other studies have shown that belly fat, not subcutaneous fat, has been linked to an increase risk for heart disease and diabetes. The UCORC study also found that those participants in the fructose group had higher total cholesterol and LDL or "bad" cholesterol levels, in addition to greater insulin resistance; symptoms which are consistent with metabolic syndrome, while the glucose group did not.

Both sucrose and HFCS are used as sweeteners. It is estimated that from 1966, when HFCS was first introduced, to 2001 HFCS now accounts for 55% of the sweetener market. The average person in the United States consumes 62.6 pounds of HFCS each year and when combined with sucrose that amount increases to 147 pounds. From cereals and breads, to spaghetti sauce, to baked beans, to frozen dinners, almost every processed food made contains sucrose or HFCS.

The Ingredient List of processed foods shows all the ingredients in the order of amount found in the food. If sucrose and/or HFCS are listed as one of the first ingredients on the list, they are major ingredients in the product and the overall sugar content will be higher. Four grams of sugar (listed on a product label) is equivalent to one teaspoon of sugar and 16 calories. This is bad in food, especially for diabetics and people trying to lose weight. You unwittingly put into your body the very thing that will prevent you from meeting your goals of healthy nutrition and healthy living.

In the beginning sucrose and HFCS were put in foods to improve the taste of processed foods. Unfortunately, sucrose and HFCS do two things, they fill you up faster and they metabolize in your system rapidly so you feel hungry again sooner and eat more. Manufacturers of these processed goods have you, the consumer, right where they want you. They know that you will now buy more of their products to satisfy the need for the comfort you find in their foods. I tell people that if you consume products with sucrose or HFCS you might as well put a bag a real sugar on your plate and eat away. Any thinking person would not do this. Yet you do it on some level when the majority of products you consume contain sucrose and/or HFCS. If you think about it in these terms then you have a better idea of why you need to limit processed foods that contain these highly refined sweeteners.

Basically, all processed sugars supply empty calories to the body and have little to no nutritional value. Only sugars found naturally in foods, such as "fructose" (which contains "levulose") in fruit, "lactose" in milk, and sugar found in unrefined honey produced from nectar by bees, are natural substances with some nutritional value. The source of the sugar will determine how fast the sugar is absorbed into the bloodstream. Whole foods, such as fruits, containing natural fructose and fiber will release sugars slowly into the bloodstream during digestion. While processed foods that contain little fiber and mostly refined sugars and HFCS, such as baked goods, soft drinks, and fruit beverages, will release these sugars rapidly. Since many whole foods, especially fresh fruits, contain natural sugars, the key is to avoid adding "refined" sugars and additional calories to what you prepare. Natural sugars are not what you need to avoid, refined and processed sugars are. For the most part, I try to err on the side of healthier choices by using products that are in their natural whole state, using any sweetener occasionally and in moderation, and opting for sugar-free or no added sugar products.

Some organic foods use evaporated cane juice instead of high fructose corn syrup. Of the cane variety, only evaporated cane juice is "raw" natural sugar. Although evaporated cane juice is essentially a sugar, it is a minimally processed sugar. Therefore cane juice retains more of the nutrients found in sugar cane. Even so, I will use products with cane juice very sparingly. All natural maple syrup is also a sugar that is minimally processed and can be used as an alternative to refined white sugar. As with evaporated cane juice, this is a sugar and should be used sparingly, as well.

There are many new sugar substitutes or artificial sweeteners on the market, and the list is constantly growing. That is why it is important to keep up with the current and changing information on sugar substitutes. There are currently five low-calorie, non-nutritive sweeteners approved by the U. S. Food and Drug Administration (FDA); Acesulfame-K, Aspartame, Neotame, Saccharin, and Sucrolose. Acesufame-K's common brand names are SweetOne, Sunette, Sweet & Safe, and Ace-K; Aspartame's are NutraSweet, Equal, and others, Neotame currently does not have a common name, Saccharin's are Sweet 'N Low, Sweet 'N Low Brown, Sugar Twin, Necta Sweet, Hermesatas, and others, and Sucralose's is Splenda. Each of these sweeteners has its own chemical makeup, which changes the level of stability depending on the way each is used in cooking and baking. Many times, different combinations can be used to determine the amount of sweetness, bulk or texture, or both; while keeping the calories low. The FDA states that the consumption of these sweeteners is safe, as long as you do not consume more than is recommended.

A newer sugar substitute is sugar alcohol or "polyol." Although, called sugar alcohol, this type of sugar substitute does not contain sugar or alcohol. This "polyol," is actually a carbohydrate, has a chemical structure which partly resembles sugar and partly resembles alcohol. The common names for sugar alcohol are Sorbitol, Manitol, and Xylitol. Some of the newer versions are called Isomalt, Erythritol, Lactito, Maltitol, hydrogenated starch hydrolysates (HSH). Sugar alcohols can be used cup for cup in place of table sugar; provides the same bulk or texture and is half as sweet as table sugar with half as many calories. Some sugar alcohols, such as sorbital and xylitol, occur naturally in certain fruits and other foods. Both the World Health Organization (WHO) and the FDA consider polyols safe for human consumption.

There are several known benefits of sugar alcohols over sugar; sugar alcohols do not promote tooth decay, sugar alcohols produce a lower glycemic response than sugar, and most sugar alcohols have fewer calories than sugar. Although sugar alcohols do not fully digest and are poorly absorbed by your body, this is why it is better than sugar. Unfortunately, because sugar alcohol is poorly absorbed by your body, this can create a laxative effect. So it is imperative that you wean yourself with small amounts at first and gradually build up the amount you consume. If you find the use of sugar alcohols to be problematic, then it may be necessary for you to make other choices in which sugar substitute you may want to incorporate into your eating style.

The latest trend in sugar substitutes is agave syrup, which is also called agave nectar. These agave sweeteners are being advertised specifically as "diabetic-friendly," "raw," and a "100% natural sweetener." Many nutritionists will agree that the agave plant has a fructose that is a slow-releasing carbohydrate; and agave nectar has low glycemic index (GI) value, which is therefore an excellent sugar substitute, especially for diabetics. In comparing the GI values for table sugar at 68 GI, honey at 55 GI, and agave sweeteners at 11 to 19

GI, it may appear that agave is a better choice. What this GI means is that agave raises blood sugar slower than table sugar. Agave is one-third sweeter than table sugar, so you would use less; and keeps your sugar cravings at bay for a longer period of time, which allows you to use it as energy versus storing it as fat. For many, agave is becoming the sugar substitute of choice.

Many health food stores and health-conscious people swear by agave nectars, syrups, and sweeteners. The agave plant contains phytochemicals, saponins and fructans, which are associated with antimicrobial, anti-inflammatory, and immune-boosting capabilities. One of the fructans, the inulin, is a natural plant sweetener which has an extremely low impact on blood glucose levels. Compounds from the agave plant are believed to have the potential to treat colon diseases, such as irritable bowel syndrome. The agave plant also has high amounts of protein-building amino acids and alkaloids. Although, research has shown that minimally processed agave products may provide nutrients and may even prevent disease, all agave nectars or syrups are not made equally.

Some agave products are neither a raw nor a 100% natural sweetener. Multiple sources state that the principle makeup of agave is starch, which is a carbohydrate. And unfortunately, this is not a healthy nutrient-dense carbohydrate, but a simple calorie-dense carbohydrate. In order to produce the nectar or syrup, the agave starch is converted into a free or unbound refined fructose. Through a refining, clarifying, and heating process, this chemically alters and filters the agave starch. So then, the final agave sweetener product is neither "raw" nor "100% natural."

Agave nectar and syrup is available in two colors, light or clear and amber. The main difference between the two colors is what happens during the processing of the product. If the product is cooked too long on a high heat of over 140 degrees or "burned," it darkens and is then designated as amber. Therefore, as a final product, agave sweeteners are both highly processed chemically refined fructose. Lastly, this refined fructose in both the agave nectar and agave syrup is much more concentrated than is found in HFCS.

As I stated earlier, the liver converts fructose into the chemical backbone of a triglyceride. Because of my ongoing problems with high triglycerides, I am personally hesitant about using agave nectar and syrup. But, ultimately it is up to you, as an individual, to make your choice.

Lastly, I want to discuss cow's milk, because of the "lactose" or milk sugar. All types of milk contain approximately the same amount of lactose per serving and it is only the amount of fat that differs. Although, drinking milk is a healthy alternative, one needs to be aware of how drinking too much can have an adverse effect. Although my mother gave up whole milk years ago and switched to reduced fat or 2% and low-fat or 1% milk, even these types of milk were bad for her. Milk was one of the foods that caused her average fasting blood glucose level to spike. For many years her A1C test results remained high at about 8.5%—10.0%. The A1C test measures a protein marker in the blood. This test reveals how much sugar (glucose) has attached to the hemoglobin in your red blood cells over the past two months. This tells the doctor immediately whether or not a diabetic is controlling blood glucose levels. The normal "in-control" level is below 7.0%, although most doctors want to see this number at 6.5%. At first, I thought my mother's doctor was setting an unreasonable goal, of 7.0%, for her. After looking closely at what she was eating and drinking and the serving sizes, I had a hunch that her milk consumption was the problem. Once she controlled of amount of milk she drank daily in her diet and followed my dietary plan, her A1C level dropped from 9.1% to 7.6% in only four months and on her next visit six months later her A1C dropped to 7.1%. She added a calcium citrate supplement to her diet and also got additional calcium from other natural and healthy sources, such as broccoli and spinach.

3. Limit Red Meats

Although red meat is an excellent source of protein, it is not the only source of protein. Protein is comprised of a large group of foods which includes: poultry, fish, game meats, dry beans or legumes, soy and soy products, eggs, and nuts.

Although red meats are a good source of protein, they are unfortunately high in the wrong kind of fats—saturated. Many people get confused with fats and look at fats as if they are only one thing—oils. This is not true and this is why you need to understand what and how to tell the difference between the various types of fat. Saturated fats are solid at room temperature and are mostly found in animal products, such as meat and butter. These fats may raise the cholesterol level in the blood, so no more than 10% of your total daily calories should come from saturated fats. One way to easily recognize saturated fats is to think about some meats that are traditionally part of your diet and ones that you may cook. Take, for example, sliced bacon or a beef hamburger. The white marbled parts that are found throughout any cut of meats are the fat. After you fry either one of these, you are left with a thick liquid fat in the pan. As this fat cools, it begins to harden slightly and becomes solid. This is the saturated fat in animal products. Although, much of the saturated fat may drain from the final cooked product, there is still saturated fat that remains in the food you consume.

While these animal products provide a necessary protein, they also contain cholesterol. Saturated fat and cholesterol are often found together in foods. Dietary cholesterol has been shown to raise blood cholesterol levels. Newer studies are now showing that dietary cholesterol raises blood cholesterol at a lower degree than once thought and this level is still at a lower level as compared to saturated fat. However, high levels of cholesterol are being linked more closely to coronary heart disease, which is a major factor in having a heart attack. If you limit the amount of saturated fat in your diet, then you will limit the amount of dietary cholesterol.

Although all meats contain saturated fats, red meats have a much higher amount than what is found in pork and poultry. In comparing cuts of meat, three ounces of lean sirloin steak has 4.1 grams of saturated fat, three ounces of lean pork loin has 4 grams of saturated fat, and three ounces of skinless chicken breast has 0.9 grams of saturated fat, while three ounces of skinless turkey breast has 0.2 grams of saturated fat. In comparison, fish is lower in total fat and saturated fat than red meat and poultry. While some fish is high in fat, this fat is mostly omega-3 fatty, which is a polyunsaturated fat, not a saturated fat. Although, some fish is high in cholesterol, because it is lower in saturated fat, this makes it a heart-healthy choice.

This rule was the easiest for me to incorporate because I was never a "red meat" carnivore, as many Americans seem to be. When dining out at a restaurant or preparing meals at home I almost always choose chicken, turkey, or fish. Red meat always made me feel heavy and overstuffed. For hours after a meal that included red meat, my stomach would feel as hard as a rock. Personally, poultry and fish have always been more flavorful and versatile. Also, I never felt overly full after eating meals with any type of poultry or fish. For example, I use chicken and turkey in everything from fajitas and tacos, to soups, stews, and salads.

If you must eat red meat, then go for the better cuts. I have a family recipe that calls for one pound of ground beef. Before my non-diet, I used to buy the lowest cost ground beef, which had a lean to fat ratio of 86/14. Now I will buy the leaner ground round, because according to the Nutrition Label, the lean to fat ratio is 98/2. On special occasions, if I make my family recipe that calls for ground beef, I will always use the leaner beefs or substitute ground turkey. By selecting better leaner cuts of red meat, I now have a better reason to not deny myself foods I used to enjoy. And I still adhere to portion control. I use the same logic when picking cuts of pork for special occasions. My husband has a red chili stew that uses pork meat. Now we buy a leaner cut of pork, roast it, and make sure to remove and discard the fat after the roast is cooked and before we add the shredded pork to the stew. It is a matter of choice of cut—leaner—and preparation—baking, broiling, or grilling. Other times, I will also replace chicken in my green chili stew and turkey in my red chili stew. This helps to lower the amount of saturated fats in the dish, making it a healthier choice. This also extends what I can include in my eating plan by stretching the ideas for meals.

Many people do not even realize that dry beans or legumes, eggs, and nuts are in the protein food category. Although these are not a complete protein, as meats, they are still a viable choice to make instead of meats. Also, beans and legumes do not contain cholesterol and are high in fiber. Many times by adding dry beans or legumes into your recipes, you can accomplish two things at once; this enables you to reduce the amount of meat, poultry, and fish you consume, so that you can lower the amount of saturated fat you consume, and by adding more dry beans or legumes and nuts into your eating plan, you can increase the amount of fiber.

Nuts are a good source of non-meat protein and do not contain cholesterol. Although, nuts are high in fats, they are the healthy monounsaturated and polyunsaturated, and are high in calories. Nuts come in a large variety and many can be used in dishes, such as stir-fry and curry. By adding this non-meat protein, you can make a satisfying vegetable dish that does not need meat, poultry, or fish. Lastly, peanuts are higher in protein than dairy products, eggs, fish, and even many cuts of meats. This makes 100% natural peanut butter, which does not contain any sugar additives or added salt, an excellent choice for an afternoon sandwich, instead of processed lunchmeat.

Another alternative to consuming any type of meat is the use of soy and soy-based products. Soy is an excellent source of protein, has a healthy mix of fats and contains no cholesterol. Soy also provides vitamins and minerals and contains phytonutrients, specifically phytosterols and phytostanols, that can help reduce the LDL "bad" cholesterol. By simply replacing meat with soy you can reduce the amount of saturated fats you consume. Once again, you can become a more creative cook by trying new recipes with soy or by experimenting with your favorite recipes by substituting soy. Other than tofu and miso, I am out of my element with the majority of soy-based products. However, I am still trying to be creative with soy.

4. Eat the Right Fats

Not all fats are oils, but all oils are fats. This is a tricky rule because the right fats, the "good" fats, are not in just one category. Because all fats are high in calories and because you do need some fat in your diet to maintain a healthy body, trying to get the healthiest balance can be a challenge.

I have already discussed the "wrong" or "bad" fat, saturated fat, in the preceding rule on limiting your consumption of red meat. I now want to discuss the "right" or "good" fats. Basically, there are two kinds of "good" fats—polyunsaturated and monounsaturated. Polyunsaturated fats decrease cholesterol, while monounsaturated fats decrease the LDL "bad" cholesterol and, at the same time, leave the HDL "good" cholesterol alone. Polyunsaturated fats are broken down into two classes: Omega-3 fatty acids and Omega-6 fatty acids, which are both essential fatty acids. Omega-3 fatty acids can be found in many foods, such as salmon, sardines, tuna, canola oil, and walnuts. Omega-6 fatty acids can be found in corn and soybean oils and a variety of nuts. Monounsaturated fats can be found in many foods, such as avocadoes, canola or olive oils, a variety of nuts, and peanut butter.

Many products have "hidden fats," trans fatty acids/trans fats. Trans fats are a second "bad" fat (saturated fats being the first). Trans fats are made by converting unsaturated "good" fats into saturated "bad" fats. Trans fats are man-made fats. Trans fats are also known as (partially) hydrogenated oil. Wherever there is hydrogenation of oils of any kind, there will be trans fatty acids present. There is increasing evidence that trans fats may increase blood cholesterol more than regular saturated fats. You should avoid products that contain trans fats and/or (partially) hydrogenated vegetable oils and try to use products that are lower in saturated fats. Once again, it is important to read the label.

I found that my problem was one of assuming that low fat or fat free was good, regardless of the product. Unfortunately, low fat and fat free does not always mean sugar-free or low calorie. Many products that are low fat and fat free can contain high fructose corn syrup, which is sugar. For example, I would purchase fat free salad dressings, assuming I was doing the right thing for my health. Then I read the label and saw the grams of sugar per serving. I learned an important lesson and I now use regular dressings with the "right" oils, but not as liberally as before.

Try to use only 100% canola oil, olive oil, soybean oil, or walnut oil when cooking, as these oils are lower in saturated fats. You may even want to try less commonly used oils, such as linseed/flax oil, grapeseed oil, or safflower oil. Butter, shortening, lard, or margarine are higher in saturated fats and should be used in moderation, if used at all. There are numerous margarines that do not contain trans fats and/or hydrogenated vegetable oils. Because my husband cannot consume butters or margarines which contain milk, he opts to use any of the *Earth Balance* organic vegan spreads. You may want to substitute any of the new zero trans fats, cholesterol-lowering margarines that are now available. When I bake and the recipe calls for shortening, I use an organic all vegetable shortening, which contains no trans fats. My husband has practiced and altered some of his bread and cookie recipes so that he can use 100% canola oil or all vegetable shortening. It is all a matter of being creative and knowing your recipes.

There are many foods that contain omega-3 fatty acids, which are a component of good fat. Omega-3 fatty acids are found in various foods, such as fish (salmon, sardines, tuna, trout, etc.) and legumes, walnuts, or soy products. Also, dark leafy vegetables, such as spinach, have small amounts of plant-derived omega-3 fatty acid. What I found difficult to incorporate in my diet was more fish, although fish is a good source of omega-3 fatty acids. I love the typical fish foods: tuna, shrimp, crab, and some types of white fish. But to eat fish regularly proved to be a test of how creatively I could prepare it. Certain fish are now my personal favorites: salmon, tilapia and freshwater perch. And I found one trick that lessens the fishy taste and smell. I know it sounds silly, fish without the fish taste and smell. I cut fresh rosemary and (after rinsing it) I place it on top of the fish fillets with minced garlic, cover and bake or steam. In preparing meals, I try to use common sense and use good fats whenever possible. This is where your creativity is crucial when preparing meals.

Avocadoes are good for two reasons: they are high in monounsaturated fats and also contain no cholesterol. Spinach, while it contains many other more important nutrients, also contains a little plant-derived omega-3 fatty acid. I use both avocado and spinach in salads and in fajitas or tacos. Because avocadoes are high in calories, I make sure to eat them in moderation. Eating nuts daily also is a way to increase healthy dietary fat and nuts provide a lot of additional health benefits. As mentioned earlier, nuts, especially walnuts, are a good source of omega-3 fatty acids. For breakfast, I will add chopped walnuts and blueberries to my oatmeal or pecans to my whole-wheat or buckwheat pancakes or crepes. Sometimes between meals if I am feeling a little hungry, I eat a handful of mixed nuts.

Common Sense and Your Own Rules

For the rest of the eating plan, I used common sense and continued to eat whole grains, beans, vegetables, and fruits. These are no-brainers in any healthy diet. So I don't feel the need to tell you that you need to eat more whole grains, because they are an excellent source of fiber and protein, and they are also lower in calories. I won't tell you over and over that you should have beans, because they are an excellent source of protein, fiber, B vitamins, etc. I won't say endlessly that you should have 3 to 5 servings of vegetables every day, because they are an excellent source of the vitamin C, beta-carotene, etc., or that you should eat tomatoes every day, because they are an excellent source of lycopene, vitamin C, lutein, etc. I won't carry on about the fact that you should have at least 2 to 4 servings of fruits, especially berries every day, because berries are an excellent source of polyphenols, carotenoids, fiber, vitamins C and E, etc., or that you should start your day with a glass of high pulp orange juice, because it is an excellent source vitamin C, fiber, limonene, etc.

For many people, the talk about fruits, vegetables, beans, whole grains, and lean meats may sound similar to various diet/weight loss plans and dietary recommendations and the foods listed in *Super Foods Rx*. But how my "I'm not on a diet" is different is that in addition to my four basic rules, you must come up with the rest of your "diet" according to your traditions, cultures, and personal preferences. What is typical for me may not be typical for you. Only you know what you like and what you and your family will eat. You need to be able to develop your own personal healthy way to eating better.

In my husband's tradition, for Ghost Supper blackberry and pumpkin pies are a requirement. We make our special whole-wheat pastry flour pie crust, with oat bran added to the dough to keep the crust softer. In the past, he typically roasted a turkey with a seasoned white bread stuffing. Now, his basic stuffing is made with 100% whole-wheat sugar-free bread, that we cube and toast in the oven. We used to make mashed or baked (white) potatoes, but now bake sweet potatoes. He makes his homemade version of "Indian bread" that his mother taught him, which is very similar to the Native breads of the southwest. Once again, he substitutes regular white flour with 100% whole-wheat flour and oat bran. He also uses 100% canola oil or an all vegetable organic shortening instead of lard or regular shortening. We still have the traditional corn soup and wild rice, with no changes. As I said, he made substitutions in preparing some traditional meals, but kept the main ideas intact. We still honor our traditions, just with a few changes in preparation.

In my culture, pinto beans (especially refried), white rice, and tortillas are a staple. If you don't serve one of these at every meal, you have committed a major sin! Twelve rosaries may not save your soul. What I change for my diet is instead of refrying beans in oil (although I could refry in canola oil); I drain the canned beans and replace with a little tap water and bring to a full boil, then mash the beans to a consistency I prefer. This is my version of refried beans without the added fat. Sometimes I add seasonings to change the flavor of the beans. I also replaced regular white rice with brown rice. Likewise, I replaced regular white flour tortillas with either 100% whole-wheat flour or corn tortillas. These are easy and healthy replacements to make and without radically changing what I would usually eat.

Numerous sources, including my doctor, state that aging women should eat more soy, because as we age our bodies need the nutrients soy provides. Soy is beneficial in preventing bone loss and has shown some success in reducing both the intensity and occurrence of hot flashes in perimenopausal and postmenopausal women. Although I am postmenopausal, I cannot bring myself to eat soy every day. I have no problem ordering and eating tofu when I eat at a restaurant, but don't make me drink soymilk or bake with soy flour. I tried it and didn't like the results. However, when preparing stir-fry, I will add tofu. Also, I actually enjoy a bowl of miso, with freshly shredded cabbage and green onions.

How to Shop for Healthy Foods

Once I developed my rules for healthy eating, I needed to ensure that everything I purchased naturally fell into these four categories. At first I believed that this would be difficult. But, in fact, this turned out to be relatively simple and more about using common sense. It also required that I pay more attention to the little details that many people forget to use. As in Step Two, regarding health literacy, one needs to become "food literate," as well. These four rules will show you how to become more food literate and how to keep increasing your food literacy.

Becoming food literate is not as hard as it seems. There are basic things about food that you already know, whether or not they are good or bad. We know that fresh fruit and vegetables are better than that slice of apple pie or the double chocolate cake. In general, most people already know many things about foods, but we choose to ignore what we know because we have this need to not deprive ourselves of the foods that bring us comfort. We want our comfort foods. We need our comfort foods. But, if you have started following the Four Rules of Eating, then you have begun the process of changing your eating habits for the better. The next natural step is to change your shopping habits.

Four Rules of Shopping

1. Read the Labels

Yes, you can do this, turn the package over, rotate the can, do whatever is necessary to find and read the labels. You need to find, read, and understand the Ingredients List and the Nutrition Facts Label. At first, you will be shocked to find what is actually in many foods. Going through this process the first time is numbing for some people. We want to have this immense trust that major food companies and corporations wouldn't knowingly make or sell something that was in some way bad for us. Unfortunately, this is more false than true. We, as consumers, must face the fact that we live in a consumer driven capitalist society in which many companies and corporations value profits and satisfying the needs of their board members over everything else. Also, to be fair, the average consumer will only want to purchase the easiest, fastest, and most affordable products available and do not invest the time to ensure that the product they purchase is of the healthiest and highest quality. To show the importance of reading both the Nutrition Facts Label and the Ingredients List, I will look at several changes made in the processing of foods. Some of these changes have been in effect for some time, while others are more recent.

Two popular additives; high fructose corn syrup, which enhances the taste and flavor of processed foods, and (partially) hydrogenated oils, which extends the shelf life of products, in large amounts are not healthy for consumers. Focusing on the additive which almost every single manufacturer infuses into almost every single product they produce—High Fructose Corn Syrup (HFCS).

The major exceptions are foods made specifically for diabetics that replace HFCS with sugar substitutes, such as sucrolose and sugar alcohol, and organic foods, which use natural sweeteners, such as evaporated cane juice and molasses. But as stated earlier, even foods with sugar substitutes and natural sweeteners should be used in moderation.

In the beginning, adding sweeteners was an innocent step manufacturers took in the processing of foods. At first, sucrose was added to enhance the flavor of processed foods. In 1966 sucrose held 86% of the sweetener market. In the 1980's when manufacturing methods improved, there was a sharp increase in the production of HFCS. One processing advantage HFCS has over sugar is because it is a thick liquid it mixes more readily into any product. It also proved to have two major economic advantages for manufacturers, as well. First, when the price of sugar rose, HFCS proved to be a cost-saving alternative. By the pound, HFCS was far cheaper than sugar. Second, HFCS is much sweeter than sugar, so manufacturers use less. Since millions of pounds of sugar were used by manufacturers annually, the savings proved to be too good to pass up. As processed foods became more and more popular it was just a natural step to add this sweetener to everything processed. This allowed companies to keep their profits higher. By 2001, HFCS had 55% of the sweetener market.

Second, the "low carb" fads, created by the Adkins and South Beach diets to name a few, have caused "low carb" dieters to identify and target white flour and white flour products as a food source to avoid and also opted for the inclusion of the "good" fats (oils) in their diet. This, in turn, caused sales and profits of many types of these products to drop. To win back some of their previous consumers, *General Mills* was one of the first cereal manufacturers to offer "improved" "healthier" cereals that are made from whole grains, instead of white flour in all their cereal products. Many other cereal makers are following this trend by reintroducing some of their own cereals as whole grain. More whole grain and sugar-free breads are available than ever before. I have actually seen and purchased 100% whole-wheat sugar-free hot dog buns and hamburger buns.

Although this is a step in the right direction, many manufacturers still add HFCS instead of minimally processed sweeteners or no sweeteners at all. And, unfortunately, almost all cereals still contain (partially) hydrogenated oils, of one type or another. Manufacturing changes with the use, or non-use, of hydrogenated oils is coming from an unlikely source. Snack manufacturers, such as potato chips and tortilla chips, are giving their products a healthy make over. Both potato chips and tortilla chips, in almost every brand name, are now made with "natural" ingredients and contain no trans fats. So eating potato chips and tortilla chips became a little healthier, although these types of products are still high in calories. You must remember this does not give you license to eat the whole bag, half the bag, or even a quarter of the bag. Everything you need to know and follow is all on the Nutrition Facts Label and Ingredients List.

First, you have to be more aware of the terms used on the entire packaging of the product, not just what is in the Ingredients Lists or on the Nutrition Facts Label. Many manufacturers used specific terms and "catch phrases" in order to get the attention of the consumer. It is important that you have, at least, some knowledge before you make any purchase. According to the Food and Drug Administration, in looking at one serving of the product, the following will apply to the appropriate term(s):

"Calorie free" has less than 5 calories
"Sugar free" has less than 0.5 grams of sugar

"Fat free" has less than 0.5 grams of fat
"Low fat" has 3 grams or less

"Lean" has less than 10 grams of fat, 4 grams of saturated fat, and 95 milligrams of cholesterol
"Extra lean" has less than 5 grams of fat, 2 grams of saturated fat, and 95 milligrams of cholesterol

"Cholesterol free" has less than 2 milligrams of cholesterol and less than 2 grams of saturated fat

"Low cholesterol" has less than 20 milligrams of cholesterol and less than 2 grams of saturated fat

"Reduced cholesterol" has at least 25 percent less cholesterol than the regular product and less than 2 grams of saturated fat

"Sodium free" or "No sodium" has less than 5 milligrams of sodium and no sodium chloride in any of the other ingredients

"Very low sodium" has 35 milligrams or less of sodium

"Low sodium" has 140 milligrams or less of sodium

"Reduced sodium" has at least 25 percent less sodium than the regular product

"High fiber" has 5 grams or more of fiber

"Good source of fiber" has 2.5 to 4.9 grams of fiber

Ingredients List

Although the front of the packaging may have statements, such as "100% Whole Wheat" or "No Added Sugar," other additives, such as HFCS and hydrogenated fats or oils may still be in the product. Unfortunately, just reading the products packaging is not enough. For myself, I first look at the Ingredients List. I do this to ensure that the foods I buy do not contain the milk protein—casein, or any sulfite preservatives. With the exception of one sulfite preservative, sulfer dioxide, the rest are easy to spot because they contain the specific word "sulfite" in their name. These include potassium bisulfite and potassium metabisulfite, as well as sodium sulfite, sodium bisulfite, and sodium metabisulfite. I have to look for these preservatives because these are "triggers" of my husband's asthma. Next, I look to make sure that the product does not contain any added fructose or HFCS, sucrose, and/or trans fats. These are specific food additives that I avoid for my own health reasons. If the processed food product does not contain these preservatives and additives, then I need to look at what is actually in the product by reading the Ingredients List.

Reading an Ingredients List is easy, but can be tiresome. Some Ingredients Lists can have a few as one to five ingredients, while some lists can have as many as 50 ingredients. I have even seen multiple Ingredients Lists, simply because there were multiple items in the package of one product, such as a variety package of frozen egg rolls. This can be a daunting task, but I need to eliminate triggers for my husband's asthma and unhealthy additives for my health concerns. This is something I need to do in order to ensure that I am making healthier food product choices in my household.

When reading the list, there are a few simple things you need to know. Ingredients are listed in descending order of weight from the highest to the lowest amount used in the product. Under the "less than 2% of . . ." section, all miscellaneous ingredients which are less than 2% in weight are grouped together. Some of the ingredients may be 2% in weight, while others may be a little as 0.5% in weight. Also, manufacturers will place any allergy alert information directly after the Ingredients List.

While, a package may state it is "Whole Wheat" or "Whole Grain," this does not mean it is actually made with 100% whole wheat or 100% whole grain. If the product is truly 100% whole grain, then it will state on the list of ingredients "100% whole wheat flour." I remember when I first made the mistake of not reading the Ingredient List. I purchased a loaf of bread that stated it was "whole wheat, sugar free" on the front of the package. While there was no added sugar, it was not "100% whole wheat." The first ingredient was "wheat flour" and the second ingredient was "unbleached white flour." This also applies to any other product, such as fruit drinks. Many fruit drinks will state that they contain "fruit juice," but may actually contain a very small percentage of natural fruit juice. To make up for the lack of the natural sweetness in the diluted fruit juices in the fruit drink, manufacturers will add processed sugars, such as HFCS. These are just two examples of why it is important to read the Ingredients Label on any product you purchase.

Also, if the product states it is "sugar free," then it should not have any added processed sugars, but may have a sugar substitute, such as sugar alcohol or maltose. If the sugar is naturally occurring, like lactose in milk products or fructose in processed fruit products, then this type of sugar will not be on the Ingredient List. However, naturally occurring sugars will be listed on the Nutrition Facts Label as a percent of daily value under the Total Carbohydrate section. In many processed fruit products, such as jellies and jams, you may find added fructose on the list. This means that not only does the product include the naturally occurring fructose, but the manufacturer added any one of the various man-made sugar substitutes, such as HFCS. Other names for added processed sugars include: corn syrup, high fructose corn syrup (HFCS), fruit juice concentrate, maltose, dextrose, sucrose, honey, maple syrup, molasses, and evaporated cane sugar, to name a few. Because processed sugars are in almost every product, it is up to you, as a proactive and food literate consumer, to be aware of what is in the products you purchase.

Finally, you need to look for "(partially) hydrogenated fats/ oils." These are trans fats and are not a healthy choice. Many manufacturers use hydrogenated fats and oils in the product to extend the shelf life. Also, you need to look for saturated fats. Many times additives get lost in the ingredient list under the "less than 2%" section because the manufacturer does not place more than 2% in the product. Also, these ingredients do not have to be listed in order of descending weight. So, they may be listed alphabetically or by category, such as all nutrients listed after foods. Just because saturated fat and any of the class of trans fats are under the "less than 2%" section, you still need to look at the Nutrition Facts Label. This will give you the exact amount of these unhealthy saturated and trans fats and the percents of daily value are in each serving.

Nutrition Facts Label

The next thing I look at is the Nutrition Facts Label. I look at the calorie count, especially in relation to serving size, the amounts of total fats, cholesterol, sodium, and total carbohydrates, which include dietary fiber and sugars, just to name a few. I take into consideration as many aspects as possible before I purchase any products. Before you can successfully read a label, you must become familiar with a label and what to look for in a label. This is much like my second step in becoming health literate. Now, you need to become food literate.

The following are some of the basic things one needs to look for in a Nutrition Facts Label. As noted, in the sample Nutrition Facts Label of generic macaroni and cheese, there are several sections on the label that are considered to be important to review. This sample label will be referred to in discussing each of the areas on the Nutrition Facts Label.

First, there is the section which includes the serving size and servings per container. This is the one part of the label that is usually overlooked. All product labels are not created equal. What I mean by this is simple—do not assume that the serving size and servings per container on one particular product will be the same for another similar product. According to the USDA, a standard serving size is 30 grams. To be on the safe side, I measure the food out on a scale, so I know what the manufacturer considers a "serving size." What may seem like a normal and typical serving size to you may be very different to what the manufacturer has placed on the Nutrition Facts Label. I even count out tortilla chips according to the serving size listed on the label. This is why you need to know what the serving size is and why you need to watch portion control when consuming certain foods.

Using the sample label, this macaroni and cheese product has a serving size of 1 cup, with a total of 2 servings per container. This means that the entire prepared container would be 2 cups and the nutritional information on the package is based on only half of the container. If you consumed the entire container, you would be consuming twice the calories, fat, and other nutrients. Likewise, if a product has five servings per container, the information on the Nutrition Facts Label would be based on one of five servings per container. If you consumed the entire container, then you would be consuming five times everything listed on the label, including calories, fat, cholesterol, sodium, carbohydrates, fiber, sugar, protein, and all nutrients. The different standards of serving sizes from one manufacturer to another, who produce similar products, such as cereals, have led to public criticism of some manufacturers.

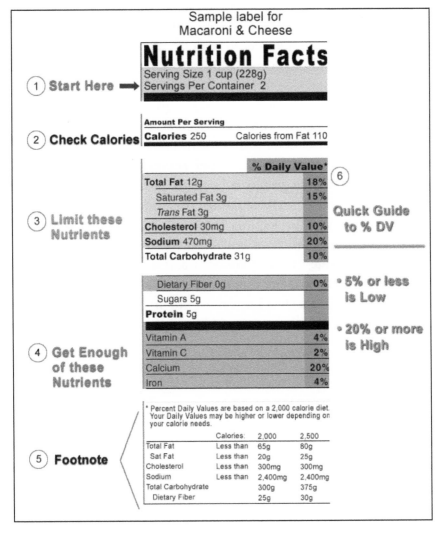

Sample of Nutrition Label

There is an ongoing battle between some manufacturers and public interest groups, which involves the advertising practices of what is termed "junk food" ads. Two public interest groups, Center for Science in the Public Interest (CSPI) and the Campaign for Commercial-Free Childhood, want manufacturers to stop advertising "junk food" to children under the age of 12. These groups define "junk food," as any product whose serving size contains more than 12 grams of sugar per serving. In 2006, these two groups filed a lawsuit in the state of Massachusetts in order to prohibit the mass marketing of "junk food" products. In order to comply with these pressure groups and to avoid a lawsuit, manufacturers agreed to no longer advertise products that contained more than 12 grams of sugar per serving.

However, in order to bypass their agreement with the various public interest groups, what many cereal manufacturers did was "to reformulate the foods to meet nutritional guidelines," thereby ensuring the amount of sugar "per serving" was under the 12 grams allowed. These groups believe that many manufacturers are using the method of "reformulating" to "fudge" the numbers and percentages on their packaging. The following chart lists, in grams, the serving size, dietary fiber, and sugar for several breakfast cereals, which are marketed toward children and adults. This example is representative of one major cereal manufacturer and shows why this first step in reading a label is the most important.

Marketed to:	Serving Size (Grams)	Calories	Calories from Fat	Total Carbohydrate	Dietary Fiber	Sugar
Children	33	132	10	29	0	15
Children	31	136	31	24	1	11
Adults	55	170	9	42	5	19

While in looking at the calories, it appears that all three have approximately the same amount of calories, with the children's cereals at a slightly lower amount. However, in comparing the actual serving sizes for the children's cereals to the adult cereal, it is almost half the amount. The serving size of 55 grams, or approximately ½ cup, for the adult cereal is twice the amount of both children's cereals; which at 33 and 31 grams are approximately ¼ cup. In order to make a fair comparison, the amounts for calories from fat, carbohydrates, dietary fiber, and sugar for the children's cereals would also need to be doubled.

In my Second Rule of Eating, No to "Ose," I wrote that 4 grams of sugar is equal to one teaspoon of sugar and 16 calories. If we look at the actual sugar content for this particular cereal manufacturer, the first children's cereal would contain 30 grams of sugar, the second children's cereal 22 grams of sugar per ½ cup serving size; while the adult cereal would contain 19 grams of sugar per ½ cup serving size. Overall, the total sugar content for the first children's cereal would be 7.5 teaspoons of sugar and 120 calories of sugar in ½ cup; the total sugar content for the second children's cereal would be 5.5 teaspoons of sugar and 88 calories of sugar in ½ cup; while the total sugar content for the adult cereal would be 4.75 teaspoons of sugar and 76 calories of sugar in ½ cup.

4 grams equals one teaspoon and 16 calories

First children's cereal:
    30 grams divided by 4 grams equals 7.5 teaspoons of sugar
    16 calories multiplied by 7.5 equals 120 total calories of sugar
Second children's cereal:
    22 grams divided by 4 grams equals 5.5 teaspoons of sugar
    16 calories multiplied by 5.5 equals 88 total calories of sugar
Adult cereal:
    19 grams divided by 4 grams equals 4.75 teaspoons of sugar
    16 calories multiplied by 4.75 equals 76 total calories of sugar

Remember that these figures are for a ½ cup serving size. Most of us, including myself, just pour the cereal from the box, without measuring. In reality, we most likely consume two to four times more than the standard serving size listed on the box. The first time you measure the cereal, you get a clearer indication as to why it is important to read the label and select cereals with lower sugar content. Below is information from the Nutrition Facts Label on two other cereal manufacturers. See if you can use what you have learned to determine which cereals are the better choices for you and your family.

Major Cereal Manufacturer:

Marketed to:	Serving Size (Grams)	Calories	Calories from Fat	Total Carbohydrate	Dietary Fiber	Sugar
Children	30	118	6	27	0	16
Children	30	118	10	26	1	13
Adults	53	188	9	45	4	20

Organic Cereal Manufacturer:

Marketed to:	Serving Size (Grams)	Calories	Calories from Fat	Total Carbohydrate	Dietary Fiber	Sugar
Children	55	214	57	37	7	9
Children	55	225	83	34	7	11
Adults	58	207	15	47	7	3

Second, is the section which includes the actual Amount Per Serving of Calories and the Calories from Fat. As the above sample indicates, the serving size per container is 2, and the amount of calories per serving is 250 calories and 110 calories from fat. If you consumed the entire container, or 2 servings, then you would be consuming 500 calories and 220 calories from fat. This would also apply to everything listed on the label, such as the Total Fat, which includes saturated fat, trans fat, polyunsaturated, and monounsaturated fat, Cholesterol, Sodium, Total Carbohydrates, which includes dietary fiber, soluble and insoluble fiber, and sugars, Protein, and all Nutrients. Also, the general rule is no more than 30% of your total calories should come from fat. So, roughly less than one-third of your total calories you consume can be calories from fat.

Third, is the section of the specific Nutrients, including Total Fat, Cholesterol, and Sodium, which need to be limited. While it is important to watch how much fat you consume, you need to remember that not all fat is bad. In looking at the Total Fat, it is more important that you reduce the amounts of saturated fat and trans fat; while also reducing the amount of cholesterol. Also, some manufacturer product labels will include the amounts of polyunsaturated fats and monounsaturated fats. As I discussed in the Third Rule of Eating, it is important to limit the amount of saturated fat and cholesterol by consuming leaner cuts of meat and replacing with poultry, and fish. Also, in the Fourth Rule of Eating, I discussed the importance of including the "right" fats, such as the monounsaturated and polyunsaturated fats. Also, sodium increases the risk for hypertension or high blood pressure. Therefore it is important that you also set strict limits in consuming products with sodium. By limiting the amounts of these nutrients, you may help to reduce your risk for developing heart disease, high blood pressure, and cancer.

Under Total Carbohydrate, I specifically look at the sugar content of nutrients to limit because of my health concerns and also because of my family history with Type 2 Diabetes. As I discussed in the Second Rule of Eating, natural sugars found in fresh fruits and vegetables are healthier than man-made, processed sugars. Therefore, it is important when reading the label you try to get products that are lower in all of these nutrients.

Fourth, is the section of the healthier Nutrients, including Dietary Fiber, Vitamins, and Minerals, that you need to get enough of. In the American western-style of eating the focus is on larger portions of animal-based proteins, such as meats, poultry, and dairy products, and less on fresh fruits and vegetables and whole grains. The majority of Americans do not get enough fiber and other healthy minerals and nutrients, such as vitamin A, vitamin C, calcium, magnesium, potassium, and iron. These nutrients may aid in lowering your risk for developing some diseases and conditions.

Many nutritionists agree that the majority of Americans get less than half the fiber their body needs each day. They suggest a goal of consuming 25 to 38 grams of fiber each day; and in order to get more easily, you should purchase products that contain at least 3 grams of fiber per serving. As an example, 4 grams of dietary fiber is 16%DV and 5 grams of dietary fiber is 20%DV. As I discussed in the First Rule of Eating, it is important to include foods, such as whole grains and fresh fruits and vegetables, which are high in fiber and provide healthy minerals and vitamins. Therefore, it is important when you are reading the label you try to get products that are high in these nutrients.

Fifth, is referred to as the foot note section, which includes the Percent of Daily Values (%DV), along with a reference chart to healthy people eating either 2,000 calories a day or 2,500 calories a day, and includes the DAILY MAXIMUM AMOUNTS for total fat, saturated fat, cholesterol, sodium, total carbohydrate, and dietary fiber. Because the grams listed under in this section are equal to 100%DV, these represent the TOTAL AMOUNTS you are allowed to consume on a daily basis. The general rule is to set a goal of consuming LESS THAN for the Total Fat, Saturated Fat, Cholesterol, and Sodium; while consuming AT LEAST for the Total Carbohydrate and Dietary Fiber. You need to remember that these amounts refer to a daily caloric intake of 2,000 and 2,500. If you consume less than 2,000 calories a day, then these amounts are higher than you need to fulfill your %DV and you will need to make appropriate adjustments.

The statement on the %DV is required to be placed on all product labels. It may be the full statement, "*Percent Daily Values are based on a 2,000 calorie diet. Your daily values may be higher or lower depending on your calorie needs:" and the reference chart from public health experts on what the %DV for a healthy person on 2,000 calories a day or 2,500 calories a day should be. However, if the package is too small, then the only information that must be on the label is "*Percent Daily Values are based on a 2,000 calorie diet."

It is important to note that the %DV information will not change from product to product, and is not specific to the product itself. These numbers represent dietary advice or dietary goals from public health experts.

The sixth, and final section, is the % Daily Value * (%DV), which are the percentages specific to what is in actually the product. These percentages, which run down along the Nutrition Facts Label, are based on the amount of recommended nutrients for a 2,000 calories a day diet. The percentages do not add up vertically to 100%. Rather, each nutrient percentage represents 100% of the daily requirements of the specific nutrient in the specific product, and based on 2,000 calories a day. This percentage allows you to quickly see whether or not the %DV is high or low. More importantly, this allows you to see whether or not you are getting enough of the "right" nutrients and too much of the "wrong" nutrients.

Do not drive yourself crazy by trying to figure out how to get to 100% of Total Fats, Cholesterol, Sodium, Total Carbohydrates, and Protein every day. A quick guide to the %DV is to remember that 5%DV or less is "Low," while 20%DV or more is "High." Lastly, remember the %DV is also based on the serving size, the same as in counting the calories and calories from fat. So, once again using the sample, if you ate the entire package you would double the %DV. Therefore, the Total Fat would be 36%DV, leaving you to eat 64% of your Total Fat allowance on all the other foods you eat during the rest of the day.

Hopefully, all of this information makes you feel more empowered when you go out to the store. Do not be discouraged about having to know all of this information when you are at the store. The important thing is for you to begin to recognize that you will need to make some changes and replace with healthier choices. As I stated in Chapter One with the Fifth Step, when you take an inventory of your pantry or cupboard, you will do this by reading the Ingredients List and the Nutrition Facts Label. So, once you get into the habit of reading the labels you will become a more skilled and knowledgeable shopper. Sure the first time, you may be in the store for a couple of hours, but then you know what you will most likely purchase on your next trip to the store. Then every trip thereafter is easier and faster. You learn to circumvent certain aisles because you know that you are not going to buy anything in that aisle anyway.

I find myself looking at other people's shopping carts and noticing their bad food choices. I feel badly about some of the choices they made for their families. After all, children learn eating habits from their parents. We wonder why our children are heavier today than we were, and why obesity, diabetes, and other diseases are on the rise. Adults and children eat more processed foods today than we did when we were growing up because there are more choices on the market and more fast foods available than ever before. Although, processed foods are fast and convenient, we still need to take personal responsibility over our food choices. That is why reading the labels is an important and critical start.

2. Generic is Fine

Many families and households, including my own, utilize a budget when grocery shopping. This is one area that I considered important because if you do not have a lot of disposable income to purchase name brands and/or organic foods, then you must do your best with what is available in your personal family budget. The main idea is to incorporate healthier foods in relation to what you, personally, can afford to purchase. So, I believe that you don't always have to buy free range, organic, or name brand. I believe that as long as you are adding more beans, fruits, and vegetables to your daily diet, you are taking steps in the right direction.

I find that my generic brands of canned pinto beans, black beans, mixed vegetables, etc. are just as good and nutritious as the name brands and most do not contain high fructose corn syrup and (partially) hydrogenated fats, also known as trans fats. I also try to purchase the sodium free or no salt added varieties of canned beans and vegetables. Since I never use these products right out of the can anyway, I figure why pay the higher price. Also, I always drain and rinse them before I use them in my recipes. When selecting generic brands, I always compare them to the name brands and to the organic brands. Although, I know that the quality may not be as high, I still read the Ingredients List and the Nutrition Facts Label. I want to ensure that the nutritional values on the generic product are consistent with the name brand or the organic brand. I compare the calories, total fat, cholesterol, sodium, total carbohydrates, and protein, paying close attention to the saturated and trans fats, dietary fiber, and sugar contents.

It is true that many studies show that organic fruits and vegetables contain more vitamins and minerals than conventionally grown food, as organic farmers do not use chemicals or pesticides. In 2007, a study by the University of California Davis analyzed the antioxidant content of tomatoes over a ten-year period. It was reported that organic tomatoes did contain higher amounts of the specific antioxidant, flavonoids. Two specific antioxidants, quercetin and kaempferol, within the flavonoids group were significantly higher in organic tomatoes than in regularly grown tomatoes. Quercetin averaged 79% higher amounts, while kaempferol averaged 97% higher amounts. However, the researchers went on to state that more research is needed to show that all organic foods are more nutritional. Although the report stated, that in this particular study, organic is overall a healthier choice, there are certain issues surrounding organic produce that are questionable. Because this particular study was conducted in a very controlled setting, this makes the findings harder to replicate among all of the real world organic farms in the United States.

However, in another study which came to similar conclusions, it was found that while organic is overall a healthier choice, there are certain issues surrounding organic foods that are questionable. First, each farm would have different conditions from one field to the next, so that the nutrients provided to the organic crop would vary depending on soil. The second flaw is that the tomato is a botanical fruit and, therefore, it would be harder to apply the findings to another type of fruit or vegetable, such as the leaves of organic spinach. Other issues to consider are where the organic produce is being shipped from. For example, vitamin C breaks down from the time it is picked, during the shipping process, until it reaches the store. Also, organic produce used in processed products change chemically and may lose some of their nutritional value. In spite of these flaws in the study and the general issues about organics, it is still recommended that if you can afford to buy organic produce, then buy organic, especially if you are consuming the skin of the produce.

The researchers in the second study went on to state, that some organic foods, such as organic crackers and organic cookies, are still no better than the regular snack foods. These researchers believe that if you are willing to spend extra money on organic foods, spend it on organic fruits and vegetables and not on organic sugars and sweets. This is one point where I disagree with them. If you buy regular snack foods, they may contain HFCS and other highly processed sugars, may contain (partially) hydrogenated fats or trans fats, and may be made from "white" processed flour. Either way, I believe that if you buy organic snack foods, then you still need to carefully limit your portions.

On occasion, I will buy only organic or name brands. For example, I purchase a dairy free dark chocolate chip product by *Tropical Source* or *Hershey's* sugar free dark chocolate mini bars, and eat them only occasionally. For a snack, I will purchase *Nature's Path* Optimum Power Cereal, with flax, soy, and blueberries or any of the *Kashi* cereal offerings, such as Go Lean, Go Lean Crunch, or Organic Promise Cinnamon Harvest. These are a few of my personal choices. And I find that when it comes to snacks and snack items, I often need to purchase organic items to avoid any unwanted additives or I need to purchase organic vegan snacks items for my husband.

Unfortunately for many people, the downside of buying organic is the higher cost. On average, organic foods are almost always more expensive. I also know some people would never buy or eat anything but organic fruits and vegetables or free-range meats. If organic or name brand brings you more comfort and security, and you can afford the extra expense, then buy organic or name brand products. Otherwise buy generic or store brand products.

3. Frozen or Canned is Fine

First of all, we can freely admit that frozen and canned foods are more convenient than fresh. I believe that as long as you make it a point to include more fruits and vegetables into your daily eating plan you cannot go wrong with whatever you choose. In most cases, fresh is usually better, but it is difficult to get fresh throughout the year. Unless you have your own garden or are willing to take the time to go to the store two to three times a week, it is difficult to ensure the freshness and nutritional quality of fruits and vegetables. Also, many shoppers will buy fresh fruits and vegetables and place them in their refrigerators for days before using them in recipes. Many of these products can lose their nutritional value because they are no longer considered to be at their peak of freshness. So, when buying fresh, make sure to use them within two to three days of purchase.

Frozen fruits and vegetables are selected and processed at their peak of freshness. This means that you can count on their consistency in both flavor and nutrition. Many times, I will splurge when a fruit or vegetable is in season and select fruits and vegetables according to the seasons when they are available. For example, during the summer months I purchase more fresh strawberries, blueberries, corn, green beans, and tomatoes (just to name a few), rather than buy them canned or frozen. And during the fall season, I will buy fall and winter squashes and zucchini. In the early spring and summer, when these are not as readily available, I will buy frozen to add to soups and stews.

As with generic brands, I always read the Ingredients List and the Nutrition Facts Label on any frozen and canned product. I want to ensure that the ingredients and the nutritional values on these products are consistent with fresh products, especially whole fruits and whole vegetables. I look at the calories, total fat, sodium, and total carbohydrates, paying close attention to the dietary fiber and sugar contents. For example, when you look at the Ingredients List on any bag of frozen blueberries, it may simply state "Blueberries." The only sugars listed on the Nutrition Facts Label will be from the natural sugars (fructose) in the fruit, which is found under Total Carbohydrate - Sugars. Although, the sugar content seems high, you need to consider that this whole food is a complex carbohydrate, which has fiber and other nutrients, and as such is a nutrient dense food.

I do not know and have never learned how to can fruits and vegetables. I am not talented enough to make a lot of typical foods from scratch. For example, I cannot make pasta sauce from fresh tomatoes, although I can make it semi-homemade from canned tomato products. Part of it is the fact that the process of making homemade pasta sauce is time consuming. However, in the particular case of the tomato, with the exception of vitamin C, it does not lose any of its nutritional value once it is canned. Also, the nutrients found canned tomato paste and sauces are more concentrated, than those in fresh. Because many of the products that are frozen or canned are done so at the peak of their freshness, I use the same approach to these products as I use with generic products. The use of frozen and canned products, particularly beans, fruits, and vegetables, is a convenient way to expand what you cook for your family.

4. Invest in a Subscription to a Health Magazine

A health magazine, such as *Prevention, Natural Health, Veggie Life*, or *Diabetic Living*, can provide updated health information from a multitude of reputable sources. If you are a member of a vitamin supplement store, such as *GNC* or *Vitamin World*, you not only receive vitamins and supplements at reduced prices, but these stores will provide their magazines free with your membership, either on a monthly or seasonal basis. The articles are in many cases short and easy to read. They are not bogged down in overly technical language, so you understand the basics of why certain foods, vitamin supplements, and exercise programs are good for you. What this will do is keep you informed on changes and will provide updated information on many aspects in diet, such as the health benefits of foods and vitamin supplements. Many of their articles report findings on studies from reputable sources, such as the Mayo Clinic or the United States Department of Agriculture.

These magazines also give you updated information and recipes for foods that you can incorporate into your diet. Many times I have found recipes that I have tried at least once and by making small changes and substitutions I have been able to expand my dietary selections. This will expand what you can eat so that you don't always eat the same thing on your diet and assist you in adapting the recipes into a meal you and your family will enjoy. These types of magazines also provide different types of exercises and exercise programs that can be tailored to your lifestyle. Whether you like to walk, run or jog, or go to the gym, you will also find many types of exercise programs you can do at gyms or in the privacy of your home.

If you do not have disposable income to subscribe to a magazine, then there are several alternatives. In most cases, these alternatives are free. First, when I go into any grocery store or pharmacy, there are usually magazine racks at the main entrance. Many stores will carry free health-related magazines that are available on a monthly or seasonal basis. I never leave any store without picking one up. This allows me to look to other sources for the latest information. It gives me other reading options, such as books, that I may want to purchase and internet websites I may want to visit.

The use of internet websites is an excellent alternative to gather information on a multitude of topics. The internet allows you to look for information that is relevant to what you want to investigate, whether it is health-related or food-related. Because topics and information changes rapidly, the internet also provides the most up-to-date information from various reliable resources. I personally use various internet websites on a regular basis. I find that I usually find new sites when I am looking into newer information that I either hear from a television news story, or read about in the local newspaper, or see on my internet home page under one of the web-based news gadgets or the "webmd.com" gadget. If you do not have access to a home computer, then I suggest that you go to your local library.

Below are some excellent health-related internet websites you can use to begin your journey to become more "health and food literate." A few are websites that deal with specific health-related issues, such as the American Diabetic Association and the American Heart Association. Others, such as WebMD and the Mayo Clinic, provide information on medical conditions, from diabetes to rheumatism to skin conditions to eye problems; provide information on medical tests and treatments of conditions and diseases; as well as provide current information on research.

Others are websites that you may find useful and interesting. The Nutrition Data website provides tools and topics, very detailed information on a multitude of food products, including a downloadable Nutrition Facts Label, with a complete nutrient breakdown, a Caloric Ratio Pyramid, an Estimated Glycemic Load for the product, and a Unit Conversion tool, which helps to convert from standard to metric or metric to standard. This particular site is extremely useful for those who are very knowledgeable in nutrition. The University of Michigan (UM) has two sites—UM Health System (UMHS) and UM Integrative Medicine Clinical Services (UMIM)—which provide information on UMHS research and the UMIM developed Healing Food Pyramid and recommendations about healthier food choices.

Another helpful nutrition-related website to access is the George Mateljan Foundation—World's Healthiest Foods. This particular website focuses on 129 of "the world's healthiest" whole foods, which are foods in their natural state. It includes information, not only on the complete nutritional value of foods, but also provides the history of the foods and recipes. Other helpful nutrition-related websites include, Produce for Better Health Foundation, which advocates the "5 a Day" program, as an easy way to get the daily recommended amounts of fruits and vegetables; and the United States Department of Agriculture "My Pyramid," who in 2005 changed its health focus to tailored dietary and exercise guidelines to an individual. Lastly, Whole Health MD is a website that merges medical and nutrition issues to provide an alternative approach to healthcare. Their website provides information from integrative medicine experts in their "Healing Centers," "Healing Kitchens," along with a reference library and current research from around the world.

Recommended Internet Websites:

American Diabetic Association
    www.diabetes.org
American Heart Association
    www.americanheart.org
American Institute for Cancer Research
    www.aicr.org
Mayo Clinic
    www.mayoclinic.com
WebMD
    www.webmd.com
Whole Health MD
    www.wholehealthmd.com
US Department of Agriculture
    www.mypyramid.gov
Nutrition Data
    www.nutritiondata.com
Produce for Better Health Foundation
    www.pbhfoundation.org
The George Mateljan Foundation World's Healthiest Foods
    www.whfoods.com/foodstoc.php
WHF Kitchen (Recipes)
    www.whfoods.com or www.whfoods.org
The University of Michigan Health System
    www.med.umich.edu
The University of Michigan Integrative Medicine Clinical Services (UMIM)   www.med.umich.edu/umim

4

The Role of Diet in Promoting Health

Common Foods and Food Groups of Diet Plans

I have thought a lot about what I wanted to say about the role of diet and eating healthy foods in my life. In order to write about the importance of foods and diet, one needs to understand several factors. I researched many different internet medical websites, read countless books and articles, and looked into different diet plans and found similar advice on foods and food groups that one needs to include in a healthy diet. The majority of dietary programs and plans promoted leaner meats, low fat dairy products and cheese, various fruits and vegetables, and whole grains. What they differed on was how and when to incorporate the foods and food groups into the final maintenance phases of their respective diets.

Because the *Super Foods Rx* book has been the most helpful to me in understanding and tailoring the way I eat to my lifestyle, I want to use this group of 14 foods as the beginning point. The super foods allow for "sidekicks" and "super sidekicks," which are generally in the same category and offer a similar nutritional profile. Therefore, the addition of sidekicks and super sidekicks will expand the foods choices to more than just the basic 14 super foods. For example, broccoli has recommended sidekicks that include: Brussels sprouts, cabbage, kale, turnips, cauliflower, collards, bok choy, mustard greens, and Swiss chard. Looking at Adkins, South Beach, Omega, and Dr. Phil's, they all include cruciferous vegetables that either includes broccoli or one of its sidekicks. Why I enjoyed trying to implement the ideology of adding and replacing the whole food system into my Four Rules of Eating was the difficulty I found in how each of these diet programs implemented the food groups within each of their phases. I was of the belief that one should never completely remove a food group from your dietary habits, because each food group supplies the body with necessary nutrients. Therefore, each food group depends on the other, in proper amounts, to supply your body with the nutrients it needs.

The Atkins' Diet stresses eating low-carbohydrate, low-glycemic-index foods, includes foods high in saturated fats, and has four phases. Phase 1 (P1) is the Induction Phase, in which the primary goal is to "induce" weight loss by changing body chemistry. This phase requires a minimum of 14 days to 6 months, in which several major food groups, such as legumes, fruits, grains, and starchy vegetables are eliminated. Phase 2 (P2) or the OWL (Ongoing Weight Loss) Phase allows for the addition of 5-grams of carbohydrates a day, more choice of carbohydrates, and mandatory carb counting. Phase 3 (P3) is the Pre-Maintenance Phase, which requires one to develop a style of eating for lifetime with foods from P1 and P2, and an increase to 10-grams of carbohydrates a day, and continuation of carb counting. Phase 4 (P) is the Life Maintenance Phase, which is a continuation of carb counting, with foods in P1, P2, and P3, to ensure you maintain optimal weight.

The South Beach Diet focuses on good carbohydrates and good fats and has three phases. Phase 1 is the Initial Introduction Phase that requires a strict 2-week cleansing period, in which several food groups, such as fruits, dairy, and grains are eliminated. Phase 2 is the Reintroduction Phase, which reintroduces certain "healthy carbohydrates" that are considered to be low-glycemic carbohydrates. Phase 3 is the Maintenance Phase in which P1 and P2 foods and food groups are continually monitored to ensure that you maintain optimal weight.

The Omega Diet, a Mediterranean type of diet plan, stresses "good fats." There are two types of "good fats" known as essential fatty acids (EFAs), Omega-3 and Omega-6. This diet tries to teach one how to bring these two fatty acids back into balance, by increasing intake of foods that contain Omega-3 fatty acids and placing a limitation of foods that contain Omega-6 fatty acids. This diet eliminates most prepared snacks, mixes, convenience foods, and reduces the intake of saturated fats and trans fats.

Dr. Phil's Ultimate Weight Solution combines behavioral conditioning with dietary objectives and has three stages. Stage 1 is the Rapid Start Plan, which is a 14-day 1,100—1,200 calorie a day period in which you eliminate all "low-response cost—low-yield foods" and eat only "high-response cost - high-yield foods" which are foods in pure, mostly unprocessed states, such as raw fruit and vegetables, vegetables cooked from raw or frozen, and certain whole grains. Stage 2 continues with "high-response cost—high-yield foods" while averaging 1,200 calories a day. Stage 3 is the Ultimate Maintenance Plan continues with the "high-response cost—high-yield foods" while averaging 1,800—2,000 calories a day.

For myself, many of these programs, were difficult to follow and unrealistic in many ways. Because both my husband and I enjoyed many traditional and culturally specific dishes, we found that some of the diet rules were very restrictive and punitive in their approach and did not address how real people like us actually ate. My husband decided to do some research into our indigenous backgrounds and found these diets did not consider many foods of our peoples. In looking into his indigenous background (Odawa—Ojibwa) he found that certain foods were considered staples, such as wild fruits, fresh fish, lean wild game, and wild rice. And in looking into my people's background, Mexican Indian, he also found certain foods were considered staples, such as beans, *chiles*, and corn. He decided to try to blend different aspects of our peoples' past dietary habits into one type of diet that could benefit both of us. And, a diet we could both follow with ease. This is how we began to set up the basics of our eating habits. Shortly thereafter, I discovered the *Super Foods Rx*. I found the book included most of our combined "staple foods" and this helped to convince me that my husband was on the right track for us to begin to eat healthier.

In recent years, I have read many other news articles related to "healthier" foods, "super foods," and "heart healthy" foods from various news sources. For example, there was a news story on the local news that featured 15 foods heart healthy foods. I went to the internet and found several 2008 articles on various types of "super foods" on WebMD. The first, which was reported from *Shape Magazine*, discussed the 15 heart healthy super foods that were shown with recommendations and changes to your dietary habits which may protect the heart and may reduce the risk of heart disease. The first is to reduce high blood pressure by eating 1) Swiss chard, 2) fresh herbs, and 3) low-fat or non-fat yogurt; the second is to reduce cholesterol levels by including 4) garlic, 5) extra-virgin olive oil, and 6) almonds in your diet; the third is to reduce high blood sugar by eating 7) barley, 8) cayenne pepper, and 9) carrots; the fourth is to lose and maintain your weight by eating more 10) broccoli, 11) oranges, and 12) lean pork; and the final change to fight inflammation by eating 13) salmon, 14) black beans, and 15) dried cherries.

In a second 2008 WebMD internet article, they reported on 9 foods that helped with weight loss and maintaining weight loss. The "Keeping-it-off Super Foods" are as follows: 1) green tea, 2) low-calorie broths or tomato-based soups, which reduce hunger and increase the feeling of fullness, 3) low-calorie green salads, unlike high fat salads which contain cheese, croutons, and high fat dressings, 4) yogurt, 5) beans, 6) water, 7) light diet shakes, which helped those people who had difficulty changing their eating habits, 8) high fiber, whole grain cereals, and 9) grapefruit.

In a third 2008 WebMD internet article, it was reported that the 5 super foods for heart health were 1) blueberries, 2) salmon, 3) soy protein, 4) oatmeal, and 5) spinach were all the focus of eating healthy to lower the risk of heart disease.

In a fourth 2008 WebMD internet article, which focused on the 9 super foods for a healthier brain, the foods that were mentioned as Super Foods to include in your diet were 1) blueberries, 2) wild salmon, 3) nuts and seeds, 4) avocados, 5) whole grains, 6) beans, 7) pomegranate juice, 8) freshly brewed tea—hot or cold, and 9) dark chocolate.

In the final 2008 WebMD internet article, the focus was on the top 10 everyday super foods, which were also identified as the easy-to-eat foods with multiple disease-fighting nutrients to help you stay healthy. These were also identified as those foods that help promote wellness and weight loss, are nutrient-dense versus calorie-dense, and are easy to include in everyday meals. The top "10 Everyday Super Foods" are low-fat or fat-free plain yogurt, 2) eggs, 3) nuts, 4) kiwis, 5) quinoa, 6) beans, 7) salmon, 8) broccoli, 9) sweet potatoes, and 10) berries.

Over the years, and especially since reading the *Super Foods Rx* book, I have noticed a trend in the majority of foods being promoted as "healthy" for your heart, "healthy" for your immune system, the "super food" for your brain, etc. These new, and ever growing, lists of "healthy super foods" for whatever the product, the promotion, or the ailment usually includes several of the super foods in Dr. Pratt's book. And in many cases, if they are not the specific super food, then they are one of the "sidekicks" or "super sidekicks." So, for myself, I believe that I have found the best general guide to my healthier eating choices.

The Importance of Making Healthier Food Choices

Regardless of which diet plan you look at or follow, they will list the foods and food groups that are common to each of the diets: fruits, vegetables, meats and beans (protein), (whole) grains (carbohydrates), dairy, fats and oils, and sweets. The most recognized food table is the United States Department of Agriculture (USDA) 1996 Food Pyramid. This original pyramid, which utilized dietary guidelines and the Recommended Daily Allowance (RDA), was developed as an educational tool to assist Americans in selecting healthy choices within their diets. Unfortunately, this pyramid was met with much controversy, especially among dieticians and health advocates. One of the major complaints about the government-sponsored food pyramid was that it was developed by the USDA, which had a vested interest in pushing various American-grown foods and crops to its consumers. By incorporating the dietary guidelines into the food pyramid, this was seen as a "political compromise" between health and nutrition experts and the food industry.

The 1996 pyramid starts with a broad base of grains and carbohydrates, to fewer servings of vegetables and fruits, to fewer servings of milk and meat. At the very top are fats, oils, and sweets, which we are told to "eat sparingly." Another complaint, in relation to the way the 1996 pyramid was presented was it gave no specific information about what was a "good" carbohydrate (whole grains) versus a "bad" (highly processed white flour products) carbohydrate, as well as what were "good" and "bad" proteins, and "good" and "bad" fats. It failed to have clearly defined "serving" sizes, so many people who ate larger portions would not count them as a multiple serving, but count it as one serving and overeat. It also made the assumption that all people engaged in a daily exercise routine, and were healthy and active. Many health advocates and researchers believed that this pyramid is partly responsible for the growing obesity epidemic our country now faces. Some critics have pointed out that since this pyramid was introduced, the number of overweight Americans had increased 61%.

So in the early 2000s, amid the growing displeasure with the food pyramid among health advocates and health researchers, the USDA decided to revise the pyramid. After consulting with nutritionists, dieticians, and health advocates, the USDA designed and released the 2005 MyPyramid Dietary Guidelines. The major changes made to the new MyPyramid were the portion sizes would now be expressed in ounces or cups rather than the generic term "serving," an increase in the amount of servings of fruits and vegetables, an increase to total fat from 30 percent of calories to 35 percent of calories, and dietary advice would be given based on three levels of activity or exercise — sedentary, low-active, and active. Health advocates hoped that these changes would bring about better health outcomes. However, some health advocates still find problems with the MyPyramid Dietary Guidelines. Because the new pyramid would include recommended caloric intake and dietary advice based on age, gender, and activity levels, many critics find that the new graphic would discourage more people with information overload. However, if you really want a starting point, then I advise you to try to use the MyPyramid Dietary Guidelines.

Although the USDA 2005 MyPyramid Dietary Guideline is the current pyramid, I will use the RDA in 1996 USDA Food Guide Pyramid to help explain the importance of each of the food groups and the MyPyramid "serving size" to clarify exactly what a serving size is. The MyPyramid is an individualized dietary guide, which still includes the basic food groups of the previous pyramid, includes a specific "serving" size in cups or ounces. However, the RDA within each food group is specifically tailored to an individual. But more importantly, the USDA's updated 2005 pyramid stresses the inclusion of physical activity as part of the pyramid and consider exercise key in maintaining a healthier lifestyle. I also included information that I found from numerous sources, such as health magazines and internet medical sites. Using this information, you need to be mindful to incorporate my Four Rules of Eating whenever possible.

Fruits & Vegetables

Fruits and vegetables are both rich sources of phytochemicals (plant chemicals) that are essential for our health. There are thousands of these natural plant chemicals and one serving of a fruit or vegetable can contain as many as one hundred different phytochemicals. The amount of phytochemicals in fruits and vegetables is unique to each individual food and work in different ways to fight disease. In order to understand why it is important to include fruits and vegetables in our daily diets, you need to first understand what these plant chemicals are, how they affect the function of our body, and why this function is important. Phytochemcials not only give each plant their color, but also give each plant their flavor. Because they also provide the plant's natural protection against predators and disease, it is believed that these can provide the human body natural protection against some diseases, as well.

The most recognizable of phytochemicals are antioxidants, which can protect cells in the human body from free radical damage. Free radicals, atoms that have unpaired electrons, attach themselves to other atoms. Not all free radicals are bad, although some can become damaged. These damaged free radicals are metabolic by-products made by our body's oxidation process, toxic substances in food, such as the carcinogens that may develop in fried foods, and toxic substances in the environment, such as air pollution and cigarette smoke. If there is an excessive amount of damaged free radicals, cellular dysfunction and disease may set in. Antioxidants have the ability to attach themselves to free radicals. These antioxidants can neutralize the damaging effects of free radicals by either interfering with the cell growth or by blocking the steps necessary for the damaged cells to grow. These antioxidants may help reduce the risk of developing many chronic diseases, certain types of cancers, and other illnesses.

Some of most common types of antioxidants are beta carotene, which is found in carrots and cantaloupes, vitamin C, which can be found in all citrus fruits, vitamin E, which is found in all dark green leafy vegetables, and selenium, a mineral, which is found in higher concentrations in mushrooms, cabbage, and brazil nuts. Because phytochemicals give fruits and vegetables their unique color, you can also easily see which antioxidant may be found in the plant by the color it is. Red fruits and vegetables contain lycopene, which is found in tomatoes and watermelon. Orange fruits and vegetables contain beta carotene, which is found in carrots and cantaloupe. Yellow fruits and vegetables contain beta cryptothanxin, which is found in pineapple and oranges. Green fruits and vegetables, such as broccoli, green beans, and spinach, contain indoles. Blue/purple fruits and vegetables contain anthocyanins, which are found in blueberries, grapes, and eggplant. White fruits and vegetables, such as onions and garlic, contain allicin.

There are several ways to categorize fruits and vegetables. First, these two plant groups can be categorized by their plant family name. Citrus, for example, includes grapefruit, lemon, orange, tangerine, lime, etc., provides vitamin C, folic acid, lutein, and zeaxanthin. Solanaceous (Solanaceae), includes peppers, potatoes, tomatoes, eggplant, etc., provides capsaicin, numerous antioxidants, and vitamin C. Cruciferous (Cruciferae), includes broccoli, cabbage, Brussel sprouts, cauliflower, etc., and provides sulforophane, vitamins A, C, and K, and numerous antioxidants. Rosaceous (Rosaceae), includes berries, almonds, apples, pears, etc., provides ellagic acid, multiple antioxidants, pectin, and vitamins C and E. Legume (Leguminosea), includes peanuts, peas, beans, soybeans, lentils, etc., provides phytoestrogens, folate, genistein, B vitamins, vitamin E, and magnesium. Allium, includes garlic, onion, asparagus, etc., provides saponins sulfur compounds, selenium, and a variety of antioxidants. Cucurbitaceous (Cucurbitaceae), includes watermelon, cantaloupe, pumpkin, squash, etc., provides zeaxantin, beta-carotene, and soluble fiber. Trying to pronounce the plant family names, categorizing the fruits and vegetables you need to incorporate into your diet, and then trying to remember why you need to do this can be a justifiable reason to shy away from trying to properly incorporate food from these two groups in your diet.

However, many dieticians and dietician organizations have come up with an easier way to eat your recommended daily requirements of fruits and vegetables. By combining all fruits and vegetables and placing them in color categories, it affords you an easy way to meet the recommended daily requirements set by the USDA. Some use the four-color category—blue, red, green, and orange—or the five-group color category—blue/purple, red, green, yellow/orange, and white. The blue/purple group includes blueberries, plums, purple grapes, raisins, purple cabbage, eggplant, etc. The red group includes red apples, cherries, red grapes, pink/red grapefruit, strawberries, watermelon, red peppers, radishes, red onions, tomatoes, etc. The green group includes avocadoes, kiwifruit, limes, green grapes, asparagus, broccoli, Brussels sprouts, green beans, leafy greens, green onion, spinach, peas, etc. The yellow/orange group includes apricots, cantaloupes, oranges, mangoes, pineapples, butternut squash, carrots, pumpkin, sweet corn, etc. The white group includes bananas, white peaches, cauliflower, garlic, mushrooms, turnips, white corn, etc. By trying to incorporate at least one to two fruits or vegetables from every color category daily, you can get the health benefits your body needs.

Whichever way you choose to monitor how much you eat daily, you need to be aware of why eating from these two food groups is important. All fresh fruits and vegetables, plain frozen and canned fruits and vegetables, 100% fruit and vegetable juices, 100% frozen fruit/juice bars, and homemade soups are considered to be "nutrient dense" foods. This simply means that in relation to the small amount of calories, they provide a high amount of vitamins and minerals per serving. Some fruits and vegetables may have a higher nutrient dense rating than others. Both groups provide important amounts of vitamins, such as vitamins A and C, fiber, and minerals. And both fruits and vegetables are naturally low in fat and sodium.

Fruits
"An apple a day, keeps the doctor away"

We are all familiar with this old saying. Yet, according to numerous sources, the average person does not come close to consuming the recommended daily requirement of fresh fruit or fruit juice. And of those that do consume products containing fruits and fruit juices, they do not eat them in their natural whole nutritious state. Instead, they consume processed fruits and fruit drinks or beverages, which contain additives, such as high fructose corn syrup. These types of processed fruits are stripped of many of their nutrients and lack the fiber found in whole fruits eaten in their unprocessed state. So, 100% fruit juice is nutritionally superior to fruit drinks or beverages. Ounce for ounce, 100% fruit juice has far more nutrients than fruit drinks or beverages, which may contain only 1% to 25% fruit juice along with added processed sugars.

Whole fruits are naturally sweet and contain natural sugars, and most do not need added processed sugars. Whole fruits are better for you than processed fruits and contain important and essential nutrients and fiber. If you must eat canned or frozen fruits or drink fruit juices, always purchase the "100% no sugar added" whole fruit varieties.

Recommended USDA daily requirements (based on a 2,000 calorie diet):

❖ Fruits and (100%) fruit juices provide important amounts of vitamins A and C and potassium and are low in fat and sodium.
❖ Eat 2 to 4 servings of fruits each day.

Examples of serving sizes:

➢ 1 medium apple, banana, orange
➢ ½ cup of chopped, cooked, or canned fruit
➢ ¾ cup of (100%) fruit juice

Because there are numerous fruits and fruit groups, I will look at several groups within this category in order to show why they are a good choice to add to your diet.

All types of berries, in general, offer dense concentrations of antioxidants, which can protect you from free radical damage. Of the top ten spots for fruit or vegetable sources high in antioxidants, berries claim four: blueberries, strawberries, raspberries, and blackberries, with blueberries considered to be the richest source of antioxidants. In blueberries, the phytochemical known as anthocyanidins, contain healthful antioxidants. Anthocyanidins not only protect the plants from oxidation it also gives the fruit its rich and deep color. It is also believed that anthocyanidins have important health benefits for humans. It is known that the metabolites of oxidation, known as free radicals, are at the root of the progression of many health-related problems, such as chronic diseases (diabetes, arthritis), many types of cancer, and the aging process. Because anthocyanidins' antioxidants are estimated to have 50 times the antioxidant activity of vitamins C and E, it is believed that they are able to protect cells and tissue from free radical damage. Not only do these berries contain the antioxidant, anthocyanidins, which help prevent free radical damage, but these four particular berries, in varying amounts, also contain proanthocyanidins, which may inhibit damaging inflammation in brain cells, and ellagic acid, which prompts cancer cells to die. Blueberries may protect your body's cells against cancer and cardiovascular disease and may improve night vision, reduce blood glucose levels, and help control the complications of diabetes. Strawberries may help to reduce blood pressure, LDL "bad" cholesterol, and the risk of heart disease and some cancers. Raspberries may help protect your body from certain cancers, especially esophageal cancer. And blackberries may also protect your body from certain cancers and heart diseases.

Citrus fruits contain a high amount of vitamin C, folic acid, B vitamins, potassium, and various antioxidants. Citrus fruits also contain flavonoids, which are found in the whole fruit. Two of these flavonoids, naringin in grapefruit and hesperidin in oranges, are only found in citrus fruits and act as both an antioxidant and an antimutagenic, which prevents cells from mutating. This is instrumental in preventing the development of cancer cells and changes that lead to other chronic diseases, such as cardiovascular disease. The high amount of vitamin C and hesperidin in oranges has been shown to help increase HDL "good" cholesterol levels, while at the same time reducing LDL "bad" cholesterol levels. Lutein and zeaxanthin may help reduce the risk of eye diseases, such as macular degeneration. Also, d-limonene, which is found in approximately 90% of the oil of the citrus zest (citrus peel), may help to protect against skin cancer. Compounds, known as polymethoxylated flavones, found in the peel of tangerines and oranges may lower LDL "bad" cholesterol levels.

When considering fruits by color, the red group (pink grapefruits, watermelons, and tomatoes) is an excellent source of a healthy phytochemical—lycopene. Of all the fruits that contain lycopene, tomatoes are by far the best source of lycopene. Although, the tomato is thought to be a vegetable, it is actually a fruit. In 1893 the U.S. Supreme Court in relation to shipping tariffs on fruits and vegetables for farmers made the ruling that tomatoes should be taxed as vegetables. In order for the body to absorb the rich nutrient lycopene, it is necessary to add some type of fat, such as olive oil, cheese, or nuts. Canned processed tomatoes have more bioavailable lycopene than raw tomatoes. By processing the tomato, the lycopene is made more readily available for the body to absorb. Lycopene prevents free radical damage, thereby reducing the risks for certain types of cancers, especially prostate and skin cancer, and helps to reduce the risk of cardiovascular disease. Lycopene also helps to indirectly reduce the risk for eye diseases, such as age-related macular degeneration.

Vegetables
"Carrots will make your eyes sparkle"

Many people have their own personal story about why they hate eating vegetables. Mine started at an early age, when upon remarking to my parents, in a rather whiny but forceful tone, that I hated avocadoes and I would not eat any. Well, at this point a few pieces were placed on my plate and I was forced to eat them. My battle with vegetables began. Although, I would eat the standard — mixed vegetables, green beans, peas, corn, and carrots — I managed to stay away from most vegetables for approximately 20 years. Then, when in my mid 20's, I went to an afternoon baseball game with friends, with the promise of a nice dinner afterwards. So, I waited all afternoon, sat through an enormous amount of post-game traffic, and finally arrived at a Mexican restaurant starving. A guacamole appetizer was ordered. When it arrived, I begged off for about 2 minutes, watching everyone at the table enjoying this dish. Finally, my hunger got the best of me and I tasted a little, just to prevent myself from fainting. Needless to say, I couldn't get enough. Because of this experience I realized that I may have misjudged many vegetables and I am now willing to try any vegetable, within reason.

Because of my experience, I now tell people don't focus on the few vegetables that you may not like. Focus instead on the vegetables that you do enjoy eating. This will get you used eating vegetables at lunch and dinner and then you can add vegetables that are in the same group as the ones you currently eat. Also, by being willing to try more vegetables, you will be teaching your children better eating habits.

Recommended USDA daily requirements (based on a 2,000 calorie diet):

❖   Vegetables provide numerous vitamins, such as A and C, folate, and minerals, such as iron and magnesium.

They are naturally low in fat and provide fiber. Select from a variety of vegetables.

❖   Eat 3 to 5 servings each day.

Examples of serving sizes:

➢   1 cup of raw leafy vegetables
➢   ¾ cup of (100%) vegetable juice

One of the more important groups of the phytochemicals in vegetables is glucosinolates, which are members of the organosulfur chemical family. Specifically in plants, glucosinolates will react with enzymes to form two key compounds—indoles and isothiocynates—which protect the plant from predator insects. Indoles and isothiocynates show the potential to have health benefits for humans, as well. In humans, these two compounds may halt the progression of many health-related problems, such as certain types of cancer by neutralizing the cancer-causing chemicals, inhibiting certain enzymes that promote the growth of cancer cells, and inducing other enzymes to aid in the dismantling of cancer cells. Also, many vegetables are excellent sources of vitamins and minerals. There are also numerous vegetables and vegetable groups, so again I will look at several groups within this category in order to show why they are a good choice to add to your diet.

Cruciferous vegetables contain high amounts of glucosinolates, enzymes that help your body that defend against diseases, especially cancers. These enzymes have shown the ability to stop the growth of cancer cells in cell, tissue, and animal models. Numerous human studies have shown that diets high in cruciferous vegetables reduced the risk for lung, stomach, and colorectal cancers, as well as reduced rates of prostate and bladder cancer. Broccoli, a cruciferous vegetable, is also a rich source of folic acid, which may reduce the risk of heart disease, prevent birth defects, and slow the onset of Alzheimer's dementia. The sulforophanes in broccoli and kale may reduce the risk of breast cancer and the isothiocynanates found in each stimulate the liver to break down carcinogens and may reduce the risk of colon cancer.

Dark green leafy vegetables should be an important part of your diet. They are good sources of vitamin A and C, calcium, and fiber. The darker green the leafy vegetable, the more nutrients the vegetable will contain. They can be eaten cooked or raw. All dark green leafy vegetables, such as spinach, Swiss chard, chicory, collard greens, kale, and mustard greens are excellent choices. In comparing a ½ cup serving of a few chopped raw greens; chicory has 90 mg of calcium, 3.6 g of fiber, and 0.8 mg of iron, kale has 45 mg of calcium, 0.7 g of fiber, and 0.6 mg of iron, and spinach has 15 mg of calcium, 0.4 g of fiber, and 0.4 mg of iron. The antioxidant, lutein, found in dark greens may reduce the risk of cardiovascular disease and stroke, reduce the risk for eye diseases, such as age-related macular degeneration and cataracts, and work to enhance the immune system, thereby preventing some types of cancer, especially stomach and lung cancer.

In the yellow/orange group: carrots, yellow and orange peppers, pumpkin, and winter squash are an especially healthy addition to your diet. The vegetables in this group are not only a good source of vitamins and minerals, they are also high in fiber and low in calories. Vegetables in the yellow/orange group provide two healthy carotenoids—alpha-carotene and beta-carotene. The absorption rate of beta-carotene differs, depending on whether the food is raw or cooked, or whether you get the carotene in the natural whole food or as a supplement. These carotenoids help to protect the body from free radical damage, which can reduce the risk of chronic diseases, cardiovascular disease and various cancers, such as lung, colon, breast, and skin cancer. Carotenoids may help to stimulate the production of detoxifying enzymes, may protect the eyes from certain diseases, such as cataracts and macular degeneration, and may protect both the eyes and skin from the damaging effects of ultraviolet light.

According to a recent study, the antioxidant, pterstilbene, in blueberries and grapes was shown to lower cholesterol in a manner comparable to popular cholesterol-lowering drugs. This antioxidant also may have the added benefit of lowering triglycerides levels (*Let's Live*, December 2004, p. 14).

New research shows that grapefruit may actually promote weight loss. Findings from a clinical trial with 100 men and women at the Scripps Clinic in San Diego, Calif., show those who included half a grapefruit with every meal lost on average 3.6 pounds over the course of 12 weeks. While, those that drank grapefruit juice three times daily lost on average 3.3 pounds (*Let's Live*, January 2005, p. 18).

Studies have shown cruciferous vegetables, such as broccoli, cabbage, Brussels sprouts, and cauliflower, contain sulforaphane, which prevents cellular changes that can lead to breast cancer and halts the growth of malignant breast cells. In test-tube studies at the University of Illinois at Urbana-Champaign, sulforaphane interrupts the cancer cells' ability to divide, which caused the cells to die (*Prevention*, March 2005, p. 78).

Pungent yellow onions contain more quercetin than white onions. Quercetin, an antioxidant, may reduce cancer risk (*Prevention*, April 2005, p. 72).

A study found that eating a large (3-cup) low-calorie salad as a first course may help you eat about 12 percent fewer calories during the meal, than those who ate no salad. While eating a small (1 ½ cup) low-calorie salad showed they ate 7 percent fewer calories during the meal over those that ate no salad (*Diabetic Living*, Summer 2005, p. 20).

Johns Hopkins University School of Medicine researchers found that sulforaphane, an antioxidant found in broccoli, protects human eye cells from UV damage. The more sulforaphane applied to retina cells before exposure to ultraviolet light, the greater the level of defense (*Natural Health*: Special Issue, Summer 2005, p. 10).

A 6-ounce daily serving of fresh-squeezed orange juice has been shown to lower "bad" LDL cholesterol and raise "good" HDL cholesterol. Orange juice supplies twice the daily requirement for vitamin C, has large amounts of potassium, folate, as well as a phytochemical called d-limonene, which aids in the detoxification of cancer-causing substances. Orange juice fortified with calcium and vitamin D helps to prevent bone loss and may reduce the symptoms of PMS (*Natural Health*: Special Issue, Summer 2005, p. 21).

A new study showed that men who ate one 3- or 4-ounce serving of watermelon or pink grapefruit a day could reduce their risk for developing prostate cancer by 82%. In comparing the diets of men diagnosed with prostate cancer with the diets of men hospitalized for other conditions, those who ate the most watermelon, high in lycopene, had the lowest risk of developing prostate cancer. Other carotenoids, such as beta-carotene and lutein, also provide significant prostate protection. It is recommended daily servings of fruits and vegetables that contain these carotenoids, such as tomatoes, pumpkin, citrus fruits, and spinach (*Prevention*, June 2005, pp. 121-122).

Researchers in Northern Ireland found that 12-year-old girls who ate high amounts of fruit had significantly higher bone mineral density than moderate fruit-eaters. The study suggested the alkaline-forming properties in fruits may help with mineral absorption and acid-base balancing (*Delicious Living*, September 2005, p. 22).

Meats, Poultry, Fish, Dry Beans, Eggs, & Nuts (Protein)

This is the food group that most people have the most difficult time with when it comes to controlling the amount they eat, and with good reason. The size portion has dramatically increased in our standard diet. What may seem like a serving size to an average person is actually 2 to 3 times larger than what is recommended by the USDA. Also, protein is not only found in meat. Many other types of foods are sources of protein. Without realizing it, many people can easily double and even triple recommended servings of protein. This happens because some people will eat from this food group every meal. For example, many restaurants extol the fact they serve double and triple hamburgers, 16-ounce burgers and steaks, half and full slabs of ribs (beef and pork), half and full baked chicken, etc. It is easy to see how many people can and do exceed the recommended USDA daily requirement, especially for meat and poultry. The 2005 My Pyramid Food Guide also includes, dry beans, eggs, and nuts in this food group.

Recommended USDA daily requirements (based on a 2,000 calorie diet):

❖ Meat, poultry, and fish supply protein, B-vitamins, iron, and zinc.
❖ Eat 2 to 3 servings each day.

Examples of serving sizes:

➢ 2-3 ounces of cooked (lean) meat, poultry, or fish (one average size hamburger, one medium chicken breast half)
➢ ½ cup of cooked dry beans or 1 egg counts as 1 ounce of lean meat
➢ 2 tablespoons of peanut butter or 1/3 cup of nuts equals 1 ounce of (lean) meat

The structure of humans and animals as organisms is built on protein, which supplies our bodies with amino acids, essential and nonessential. Essential amino acids cannot be made naturally in our body and must come from a food source, while nonessential amino acids can be produced naturally in our bodies from other amino acids. Our bodies take the protein and change it into the amino acids we need for proper functioning, to build muscle, and to stay healthy. Dietary protein is also broken down into two distinctive categories — complete proteins and incomplete proteins. Simply put, complete proteins, which can be found in meat, poultry, fish, cheese, eggs, and milk, contain sufficient amounts of all of the essential amino acids. Incomplete proteins, which can be found in a variety of foods, such as grains, legumes, and nuts, contain some of the essential amino acids. This is why it is important to include a variety of protein-based foods into your healthy eating plan. You should never depend on one category of protein. Rather, you should develop an eating style which reflects a healthy complement of several foods in the protein category.

All meats, poultry, and fish give you a complete complement of necessary amino acids and are a good source of iron, zinc, thiamine, niacin, and vitamin B-12. However, some meat, poultry, and fish that are higher in minerals may be lower in vitamins; while some may be higher in vitamins and lower in minerals. As stated above, the key for better nutritional value is including a variety of all protein sources into your diet. Excellent sources of protein can also be found in a multitude of non-animal foods, such as dry beans and nuts.

Meats

Beef

When choosing the type of beef you want to incorporate into your diet, you must look at several factors. First, you need to look at the grade of beef. Beef comes in a variety of grades. Grading, by slaughterhouses, is a voluntary service offered by the USDA. The meat is evaluated on how much marbling, the white streaks of fat within the flesh of the meat, is present. This marbling gives the meat its flavor and texture. Meat with the most marbling is given the highest rating of Prime, followed by Choice then Select. Select cuts have approximately 5% to 20% less fat than Choice and approximately 40% less than Prime. Because grading of beef is voluntary, on average 44% of the beef in supermarkets is not graded and is typically sold as Select or Choice. Second, you must consider the cut or what part of the animal this meat is from. Determining the cut of beef is sometimes more important than determining the grade. The Select of one cut may have more fat than the Choice or Prime cut of another. So, it is very important to consider the lean to fat ratio when selecting any piece of beef. Because today's breeders are crossbreeding leaner, larger cattle with traditional cattle, more breeders are grass feeding, rather than corn feeding their herds, and cattle are being sent to market at a younger age, the cattle are leaner and less fatty.

Beef is one of the most versatile meat because it comes in numerous cuts; such as brisket, chuck, flank, foreshank, ribs, round, short loin, plate, sirloin, and ground beef. Each of these cuts is then divided into a variety of cuts. For example, the chuck cut includes the chuck eye roast, boneless top blade steak, arm pot roast, boneless shoulder pot roast, cross rib pot roast, blade roast, short ribs, flanken style ribs, and stew beef; while the sources for ground beef are the chuck, sirloin, or round portions. Overall, there are approximately 300 different retail cuts. A typical meat counter, at any retail store, may display over 50 various styles or cuts of beef. The label will state where the cut of beef originated. No one cut of beef is leaner than another cut of beef, this will entirely depend on the grade assigned the beef.

Fats from meat are problematic especially if you consume more calories from fat than your body uses as energy. High levels of fat, saturated fat, and cholesterol can increase the amount of cholesterol in your blood. Beef does contain the highest amount of "bad" or saturated fats, when compared to poultry and fish. However, beef does provide some of the highest amounts of protein, iron, thiamine, zinc, and vitamin B-12. For example, four ounces of lean beef provides 64% of the daily value of protein. If you choose to consume beef then you need to put its nutritional value in the proper context of how much you actually consume each day and how it is prepared for consumption. There is a big difference between eating a lean cut of select beef that is broiled with a side of steamed vegetables and eating a triple cheeseburger, with a double order of fries. Therefore, it is important that you try to incorporate leaner cuts of meat and follow the USDA daily requirements, in order to control the amount of saturated fat in your diet.

Pork

Pork, unlike beef, has no grading system because fresh pork is considered consistent in quality. However, the USDA does inspect pork for wholesomeness. Like beef, many breeders are improving the way they raise pigs for market. What this means is that pigs are also leaner and less fatty. The fat in pork slightly less saturated than the fat in beef. Although this is promising, pork is still not as lean as skinless chicken or turkey and fish. Because pork is available in the form of fresh cuts or cured, it is important to know what types of pork are available and which are considered to be the leanest. Of the fresh cuts of pork—leg, loin, tenderloin, shoulder, and side—the loin and tenderloin are the leanest portions of pork. The loin portion, usually cut into chops, has three parts—blade loin, center loin, and sirloin. The tenderloin is the source of the crown roast and the country-style ribs. Cured pork products are bacon, pancetta (Italian-style bacon), Canadian bacon, ham, and sausages. Cured pork is high is both fat and sodium and the trend for processors is to make low- or reduced sodium and low- or reduced fat pork products. It is important when purchasing any cured pork product that you read the label to see how it is cured. For example, when purchasing a ham, look on the label for "ham with water," or "ham with natural juices." Avoid hams that have added sugars. Also, look for ham that is lean, meaning it contains no more than 10% fat by weight, or extra-lean, which contains no more than 5% fat by weight.

Pork is a good source of protein and provides high amounts of iron and zinc. It is an excellent source of B-vitamins, specifically thiamin—a B-vitamin necessary to convert carbohydrates into energy for the body and helping with the normal functioning of the cardiovascular and nervous system. As with beef, you need to select the leanest pork in order to reap the benefits of this meat. For example, 3 ounces of fried center loin pork chop is 226 calories, 14 grams of fat, 5 grams of saturated fat, and 91 milligrams of cholesterol; 3 ounces of spareribs is 338 calories, 26 grams of fat, 10 grams of saturated fat, and 103 milligrams of cholesterol; 3 ounces of cooked bacon is 487 calories, 42 grams of fat, 15 grams of saturated fat, and 72 milligrams of cholesterol; and 3 ounces of regular cured ham is 151 calories, 8 grams of fat, 3 grams of saturated fat, and 50 milligrams of cholesterol.

Game Meats

Game refers to all wild animals and birds. All game animals are classified as "red" meats. Mainly because game birds are similar to poultry (birds of flight), many consider these birds to be "white" meats. However, the breast meat of game birds is darker than the breast meat of domesticated birds, like chicken and turkey. There are three classes of game meats—large game animals, such as buffalo, deer, elk, moose, and wild boar; small game animals, such as rabbit, squirrel, and raccoon; and game birds, such as pheasant, wild ducks, and wild turkey. Most Rock Cornish hens are not game birds, but are actually young domesticated chickens. Of the large game animals, "venison," which is the culinary term, is the most recognizable. Venison is meat from deer, elk, moose, caribou, antelope, and pronghorn. When selling venison, the source of the animal must be specified. Farm-raised game species can be sold, but these farms must follow state regulations. Wild game that is legally hunted cannot be sold and can only be used for personal consumption.

Wild game animals are natural forage eaters and are more active, so their meat will be leaner, less fatty, and, in some cases, can be less tender. Game meats should be braised, cooked slowly with moist heat, or roasted with dry heat in order to keep the meat moist and tender. Although some game meat can be higher in cholesterol than domestic meats, such as beef, pork, and poultry, most game meats are lower in calories, saturated fats, and total fats. Also, game meats are higher in cholesterol-reducing polyunsaturated fats, which contain essential omega-3 fatty acids. The eicosapentaenoic acid (EPA) in omega-3 is important in reducing the risk of developing atherosclerosis, which is the major cause of heart attacks and strokes. Because saturated fats effects the blood cholesterol levels more than the amount of dietary cholesterol, game meats are quickly becoming more popular among health-conscious dieters.

The following is a chart of 3.5 ounces of selected types of domestic and game meats that shows the amount of protein, fat, cholesterol, and calories for each type of meat.

Type of Meat:	Protein %	Fat %	Cholesterol	Calories
Beef (USDA choice)	22.0	6.5	72	180
Buffalo	21.7	1.9	62	138
Moose	22.1	.5	71	130
Elk	22.8	.9	67	137
Whitetail Deer	23.6	1.4	116	149
Mule Deer	23.7	1.3	107	145
Squirrel	21.4	3.2	83	149
Cottontail Rabbit	21.8	2.4	77	144
Jackrabbit	21.9	2.4	131	153
Pork	22.3	4.9	71	165
Wild Boar (fat untrimmed)	28.0	4.38	109	160
Chicken	23.6	.7	62	135
Turkey (domestic)	23.5	1.5	60	146
Wild Turkey	25.7	1.1	55	163
Pheasant (domestic)	23.9	.8	71	144
Wild Pheasant	25.7	.6	52	148
Duck (domestic)	19.9	4.25	89	180
Mallard	23.1	2.0	140	152

Poultry

Chicken

Like beef, chicken is also graded. But unlike beef, chicken is not graded by how much fat the meat contains. Grade A chickens are meaty, well-shaped, free of feathers, and have a layer of fat; while lesser quality chickens, Grade B and Grade C, are usually sold to food manufacturers for use in processed chicken products. Like beef, not all chicken is low in fat. Skinless chicken contains half the fats of chicken with the skin. The skin and the fat layer of chicken gets approximately 80% of its calories from fat, and approximately 23%

of its calories from saturated fat. So make sure that you remove the skin and the fat layer from the chicken before preparing or eating. Also, the chicken breast or the white portion is much leaner and contains less cholesterol than the thigh and leg or the dark portion.

Chicken is also one of the most versatile meats. You can bake, broil, or fry chicken; or use chicken in fajitas, stews, soups, stir-fry, or salads. Whether you choose the dark or white portion, chicken is an excellent choice for protein and other vitamins and minerals. Four ounces of chicken is a good source of protein and provides 67.6% of the daily value of protein. And chicken supplies almost the same amount of vitamins and minerals as beef. Although beef does supply slightly more iron and zinc. In comparing the white and dark portions of chicken, 3 ounces of skinless, roasted chicken breast is 142 calories, 3 grams of fat, 1 gram of saturated fat, and 73 milligrams of cholesterol; 3 ounces of skinless, roasted chicken thigh is 178 calories, 9 grams of fat, 3 grams of saturated fat, and 80 milligrams of cholesterol.

Turkey

In the past, the majority of turkey was sold only during the holiday seasons of Thanksgiving and Christmas. Turkey is making a turnaround and is quickly becoming the meat to eat, and with good reason. Of all the meats on the market, turkey is the leanest of meats and the lowest in calories and saturated fat. Turkey is a good source of protein, vitamins and minerals. Like other meats, it is a good source of the trace mineral selenium. Selenium is an essential component of several of the major metabolic pathways, including the thyroid hormone metabolism, antioxidant defense systems, and immune function.

Like the meat of chicken, the breast (white portion) of the turkey is also lower in calories and fat than the thigh and leg (dark portion), both with and without the skin. Four ounces of turkey is a good source of protein, providing approximately 65.1% of the daily value of protein. Turkey is also lower in calories, fat, saturated fat, and cholesterol than all other meats. For example, 3 ounces of skinless, roasted turkey breast is 115 calories, 1 grams of fat, 0.2 gram of saturated fat, and 71 milligrams of cholesterol; 3 ounces of skinless, roasted turkey leg is 135 calories, 3 grams of fat, 1 gram of saturated fat, and 101 milligrams of cholesterol.

Fish

All fish and shellfish are an excellent source of protein. However, not all fish are created equal. There are two basic types of fish: lean fish and fatty fish. Lean fish contains less than 1% fat, while fatty fish contains more than 1% fat and can be further divided into two types: semi-fatty fish, which contains between 1% and 10% fat, and fatty fish, which contains more than 10% fat. Lean fish is usually a whitefish; such as cod, haddock, sole, and all shellfish. Some types of semi-fatty fish are pike, whiting, sea trout, Pollock, halibut, perch, catfish, and fresh herring. While some types of fatty fish are eel, mackerel, sardine, salmon, and tuna. Because there is such a wide variety of fish and shellfish to choose from, it is important that you at least know which type of fish—fatty, semi-fatty, or lean—you prefer to place in your diet.

Although, high in omega-3 fatty acids, fish contains cholesterol. However, with the exception of shrimp, the amount of cholesterol in fish is lower than what is found in beef, pork, and poultry. There is much debate as to whether fatty fish or lean fish are the healthier choice. Some studies have shown that lean fish is heart-healthy, lowers blood pressure, and reduces inflammation, but now newer studies are showing that eating more of the fatty fish may have a slightly better health protecting effect than the leaner fish. Both lean and fatty fish have the healthy omega-3 fatty acids. However, these "good" fats are found to be highest in fatty fish and will be higher in calories. Lean fish, lower in fat and calories, are an excellent source of high-quality protein, and have a milder flavor. This makes lean fish a tasty and healthy alternative to meat and poultry. What I suggest is that you eat a compliment of both fatty and lean fish during the week. For example, you can eat a tuna (fatty) sandwich or shrimp (lean) salad for lunch; you can eat salmon (fatty), perch (semi-fatty), or haddock (lean) for dinner. As with other meats and poultry, there is also a variety of ways to prepare fish; poaching, steaming, broiling, baking, planking, grilling, and frying.

Dry Beans

Dry beans refer to a class of legumes that are dried for storage. In the store, dry beans can be found in the dry form or cooked and canned. Dry beans are almost a perfect fat-free food. Beans are an excellent source of dietary fiber. Beans contain a higher proportion of protein than any other plant food, are a major source of complex carbohydrates, and supply a substantial amount of vitamins and minerals; which include iron, zinc, potassium, magnesium, manganese, phosphorus, and thiamin. All beans and related legumes are high in soluble fiber, which means that the carbohydrates in beans are absorbed more slowly into your body than simple carbohydrates found in foods, such as white breads. Therefore, your blood glucose levels will not spike as rapidly. Also, the fiber acts to bind with bile acids that are used to make cholesterol. Since fiber cannot be absorbed into the body, it helps to expel the bile acids from the body. Beans also contain insoluble fiber, which increases stool bulk and therefore, will prevent constipation. Although almost all dry beans are high in protein, it is still an incomplete protein. By simply adding rice or other grains, nuts, any meat, poultry, or fish, this will supply the missing amino acids. Beans can be used in the main dish or as a side dish, depending on how they are prepared.

Beans come in hundreds of varieties, and because they are an inexpensive food, they are one of the most versatile foods. Some of the most common, and therefore popular, beans are; adzuki (azuki) beans, black (turtle) beans, black-eyed peas (cowpeas, black-eyed beans), cannelloni (white Italian kidney beans), chickpeas (garbanzos, garbanzo beans), cranberry beans, fava (broad) beans, flageolets (immature kidney beans), Great Northern beans, kidney beans, Lima beans, mung beans, navy beans, pinto beans, red beans, soybeans, and split peas. Although, eating any variety of beans is healthy, I will highlight the most typical, along with their nutritional value. This will give you an idea as to why beans should be a daily part of your diet.

Soybeans, native to East Asia, have higher amounts of protein and essential fatty acids than any other legume, are a major source of fiber, and are low in carbohydrates. Soy protein is a complete protein that aids in the reduction of LDL "bad" cholesterol. Soybeans are a good source of calcium, magnesium, lecithin, riboflavin, thiamin, folate (folic acid), and iron. Soybeans can count in either the meat (protein) or dairy (calcium) category towards your recommended daily requirement. Although much of the calcium in soybeans is lost during processing, many manufacturers add calcium to soy products, such as soymilk, soy cheese, and tofu. So look for "calcium-enriched" on the label of soy products. Soybeans are also an excellent source of isoflavones, a plant chemical that has an estrogen-like hormonal effect on the body. Isoflavones are also found in soy products, such as soymilk, tofu, and tempeh.

Black beans are staple beans that are used in many Latin American cuisines, but more noticeably in both the Cuban and Puerto Rican cuisines. Many people mistakenly link this bean strictly to the Mexican culture, but the majority of Mexican cooks will only use pinto beans in their dishes. Because of its rich dark color, black beans make any dish look and taste more exotic. Black beans have one of the highest amounts of fiber of all beans. One cup of boiled black beans contains 59.8% of the recommended daily intake of fiber.

Pinto beans are one of the main staple foods of the Mexican culture, along with corn and red and green chili. Pinto beans are the most popular bean in the United States and are the most recognizable bean. This bean is medium sized and light reddish tan with brown flecks. Pinto beans like black beans have high amounts of fiber and one cup of cooked pinto beans contains 58.8% of the recommended daily intake of fiber.

Kidney beans are available in several colors, but the most

recognizable are the dark red and light red. White Italian kidney beans are also known as cannelloni beans. Kidney beans are large beans that are named for their kidney shape. They will hold their shape during cooking and absorb the surrounding flavors. This makes kidney beans a favorite type of bean to use in dishes that are simmered. One cup of cooked kidney beans contains 45.3% of the recommended daily intake of fiber.

Lima beans are available in two sizes: large Limas known as Fordhooks or butter beans, and smaller Limas known as baby Limas, which are milder tasting. As the name implies, Lima beans are thought to originate in Lima, Peru. This bean is best known for its use in a Native American dish—succotash (which also includes another Native American staple, corn). One cup of cooked Lima beans contains 52.6% of the recommended daily intake of fiber.

Split peas are really green peas that, once dried and with their skin removed, naturally split. Hence, the name split pea. Although removing the skin reduces the amount of fiber, they still provide a substantial amount of fiber, vitamins, and minerals. This bean is available in two colors—yellow and green. This bean is the main ingredient in split pea soup. One cup of cooked split peas contains 65.1% of the recommended daily intake of fiber.

What I prepare and how much time I have to prepare a meal determines which type of bean (for example; black, kidney, pinto) I will purchase and in what form (canned or dry). Although canned beans are pre-cooked and therefore faster and more convenient, there are the issues of the added sodium and preservatives. Some people may find canned beans too salty, so if available, I will purchase "no salt added" canned beans. If not, I simply rinse the beans before I cook and I do not add any additional salt. This also helps to limit and control the amount of salt in my diet.

On occasion, I will prepare beans directly from their dry state. This allows me to season the beans however I choose and gives me greater autonomy on the final flavor. I will often cook the beans in a slow cooker. I prefer this method for two reasons. First, I do not have to stay at home and watch the beans cooking and second, this allows the beans to simmer slowly and will therefore give the beans a better flavor. I often make my traditional *frijoles de olla* (pinto beans cooked in a pot) in this manner. I use an organic dry seven-bean mix to use as a base for soup in a slow cooker in which I sometimes add chicken or ham. I also purchase dry split peas and will prepare a homemade split pea and ham soup in the slow cooker.

Eggs & Nuts

Eggs

Like meat and poultry, eggs are inspected and graded by the USDA. Grading is voluntary and grades of AA, A, and B indicate the level of freshness, along with other criteria. These criteria include, the inside and outside condition of the egg, cleanliness, soundness, and the shape and texture of the shell, to name a few. Once again, federal grading is not mandatory, but the majority of eggs sold as fresh are graded. Grade B eggs are not sold fresh and usually end up in egg products.

Eggs are an inexpensive excellent source of protein. A large egg provides approximately 6 grams of protein. Also, eggs provide many B-vitamins, riboflavin, selenium, some iron, and choline. Choline is a key component of the fat-containing structures in cell membranes and is especially important to brain function and health. If a person has a choline deficiency, this can cause a deficiency of folic acid—a critical B-vitamin. One large egg contains 300 micrograms of choline, which is found in the yolk.

All of the fat and cholesterol of an egg are in the yolk. Although eggs are high in cholesterol they are not a major source of cholesterol. Some studies are now indicating that people on low-fat diets can include one to two eggs three times a week without significantly changing their blood cholesterol levels and it is saturated fats in the diet that influences blood cholesterol levels the most. The egg white is almost pure protein and is considered almost perfect because it has the balance of amino acids. If you are concerned with your cholesterol and want to limit the amount of cholesterol in your diet, then using egg whites or liquid egg substitutes, which are made from egg whites, in cooking is an excellent choice.

Nuts

Nuts are a good source of non-meat protein. However, the protein found in all nuts, with the exception of Brazil nuts, is an incomplete protein. So like beans, they need to be combined with other foods, such as rice or other grains and meat, poultry, or fish, in order to provide all of the essential amino acids. Most nuts are high in potassium and iron, are a good source of vitamin E, B-vitamins, such as thiamin, niacin, and riboflavin, and minerals, such as magnesium, zinc, copper, and selenium. Because nuts are a plant food, they do not contain cholesterol. However, most nuts are high in healthy fats—monounsaturated and polyunsaturated. Although most of the fat is unsaturated fat, some nuts are higher in certain fats than others. Some of the nuts high in monounsaturated fat are macadamias, cashews, almonds, pistachios, and pecans. While nuts high in polyunsaturated fat are walnuts, hazelnuts, pine nuts, and Brazil nuts.

Portion control is very important when adding nuts to your diet. For this reason, I consider nuts a part of the fats, oils, and sweets category and eat them in moderation. It is easier to control the amount of nuts you eat by combining them with a meal. For example I add a small handful of chopped walnuts in oatmeal for breakfast, pine nuts in a salad for lunch, almonds in a stir-fry for dinner, or even mixed nuts between meals to help curb my appetite. Since roasting can destroy most of the thiamin, in nuts, you may want to choose raw or un-roasted and unsalted nuts. Although I usually choose the roasted rather than the un-roasted nuts, I still avoid the salted varieties. Since there are a large variety of nuts you can choose from to include in your diet, I will discuss some of the more common varieties on the market.

Almonds come in two varieties: bitter and sweet. The bitter

almonds are inedible and are used to make almond oil, which is a flavoring agent for foods and liqueurs. Sweet almonds are the variety that can be eaten. Almonds are high in monounsaturated fats, the same type of health-promoting fat found in olive oil. Almonds are an excellent source of vitamin E, and contain the highest level of non-animal calcium.

Walnuts are available in three main varieties: the English (Persian) walnut, the black walnut, and the white walnut. Of these, the English variety is the most popular because the shell is thinner and easily broken; the black walnut has a tougher thicker shell and has a more pungent distinctive flavor. The white walnut is sweeter and oilier, but not as widely available as the English and black walnut. Walnuts are high in omega-3 fatty acids, which is an essential and protective fat that the body is not able to manufacture.

Pecans are higher in fat and calories and lower in protein than most other variety of nuts. Even so, 60% of the fat in pecans is a "good" fat—monounsaturated. This fat is beneficial in controlling blood cholesterol levels. Also, pecans are naturally sodium and cholesterol free and are a good source of protein, magnesium, vitamin E, and zinc.

Brazil nuts are considered to be one of the most nutrient dense nuts. They contain an extremely high amount of selenium and are a complete protein, which means that this nut contains all of the essential amino acids that are instrumental to cell maintenance and growth.

Cashews are actually the seeds that are attached to the bottom of the cashew apple, the fruit of the cashew tree. They are high in vitamin C and selenium, which is known to have anti-cancer properties. Cashews are lower in fat than most other nuts and 75% of their fat is the "good" monounsaturated fat.

Macadamias are high in monounsaturated fat. Because the oil of the macadamia nut is like olive oil, the cornerstone of the Mediterranean Diet, macadamia nut oil is quickly gaining popularity.

Peanuts are not a true nut, but are actually a legume. There are three varieties of peanuts: runners, which are used mainly to make peanut butter; Virginia peanuts, which are usually sold roasted in the shell; and Spanish peanuts, which have a reddish-brown skin and are used in candies, peanut butter, and as salted nuts. Peanuts are higher in protein than dairy products, eggs, fish, and many cuts of red meat. Peanuts also contain many of the essential B-vitamins and mineral. Also, the skin of Spanish peanuts contains a concentrated source of resveratrol, an anti-oxidant that is associated with lower risks of heart disease. When shopping for peanut butter, I always select "100% natural peanut butter" with no additional salt added.

A recent study found that almonds help you stay on your diet by keeping you satisfied longer, and thereby, prevent eating between meals. The fiber in almonds stops some of the fat from being absorbed and used by the body as calories. An empty *Altoids* tin holds about 22 almonds, which is a 1-oz and 169 calorie serving (*Prevention*, April 2004, p. 68).

Researchers found that compounds in soy bind to estrogen receptors on cells, making them unavailable to more potent hormones. Also, a soy constituent, lunasin, increases the activity of about 123 different genes in prostate cells. Among these are genes that suppress tumor growth, initiate repair of damaged DNA, and promote apoptosis, which signals the damaged cells to die before they can multiply (*Newsweek*, January 17, 2005, p. 47).

A recent study of 37,000 women found that those who ate red meat at least five times a week had a 29% higher risk of Type 2 Diabetes than those who ate it less than once a week. Women who ate processed meats, like bacon and hot dogs, at least five times a week had a 43% higher risk of diabetes than those who ate them less than once a week. The researchers believe the cholesterol in red meats and the additives in processed meats are to blame (*Prevention*, March 2005, p. 78).

People who eat a few servings of fiber-rich beans each week lower their risk for heart disease up to 22%. Beans also contain phytochemicals, including saponins and phytosterols, which lower blood cholesterol. One cup of beans provides almost one-third of a woman's daily need for iron and no extra fat (*Natural Health*: Special Issue, Summer 2005, p. 25).

Omega-3 fatty acids, found primarily in fish and some plant-based foods such as walnuts, can help you to lose weight. Researchers presented the results of a study of 20 extremely obese women (BMI greater than 40) who were on a very low-calorie diet. During a three-week period, those who also took omega-3 fatty acids from fish oil lost 20% more weight (*Let's Live*, June 2005, p. 18).

Bread, Cereal, Rice & Pasta (Carbohydrates)

When you hear that a balanced diet should include 100% whole-wheat and whole grains, many people envision a bowl of dry grass and pieces of tree bark in a bowl. This is not what whole grains are! And more importantly not what whole grains can be in your diet. In order to bring whole-wheat and whole grains into your daily diet, one needs to understand why whole grains are important. It is also important to become aware of the numerous choices within the whole grain category that are available to consumers, such as buckwheat, oats and oat bran, blue and yellow cornmeal, rye, and durum wheat, to name a few. Also, whole grain foods are not limited to flour-based types of foods, such as breads, pastries, noodles, and cereals, but include wild, brown, and specialty rice, barley, quinoa, teff, and chia.

When choosing any bread, cereal, rice, or pasta, it is important that you choose 100% whole grain, whenever possible. It is not enough to simply state that whole grains and whole grain products can play a significant role in your diet. It is important to understand why whole grains are important nutritionally. Like fruits and vegetables, whole grains contain valuable phytochemicals. These phytochemicals are found in the bran and the germ of the grain. These parts of the plant provide not only fiber, but other important nutritional elements, such as resistant starches, vitamins, and minerals, as well. Some phytochemicals found in whole grains include phytoestrogens, tocotrienols, lignans, saponins, and caffeic, ellagic, and ferulic acids. These are shown to reduce the risk of developing cardiovascular disease, some types of cancer, and other chronic illnesses. For example, ferulic acid, which is an important and potent antioxidant, is able to attach to and remove damaged free radicals and inhibit the formation of cancer promoting compounds. This particular antioxidant has been shown to prevent colon cancer in animals and in other experimental models.

Eating whole-wheat and whole grains have been found to significantly reduce your risk for heart disease and diabetes. Refining grains strips away nearly all of the fiber and phytochemical content. This is why it is important to incorporate 100% whole grains into your diet. Although, the following USDA recommendations are considered important for good health, it is found that fewer than one in ten people consume the recommended daily requirement of "whole grains."

Recommended USDA daily requirements (based on a 2,000 calorie diet):

❖   These foods provide complex carbohydrates (starches), which are an important source of energy, especially in low-fat diets. They also provide vitamins, minerals and fiber. To get the fiber you need, at least half the grains you eat each day should come from "whole grains," such as whole-wheat bread and whole grain cereals.
❖   Eat 6 to 11 servings each day.

Examples of serving sizes:
➢   1 slice of bread
➢   1 ounce of ready-to-eat cereal
➢   ½ cup of cooked cereal, rice, or pasta

Bread, Cereal, & Pasta Whole Grains

Once I began to make changes in my diet, I found it easier to eat only whole-wheat and whole grain foods. First, I found that the refined processed grains were less tasty, had less texture, and most importantly were less filling. Second, I found that in processed grains and, in general, processed foods there were more unnatural additives that made them a less healthy choice. So, it became obvious and less confusing to just select 100% whole-wheat and 100% whole grains. The following are just a few, from a large and ever expanding variety of grains, I will highlight in this section.

Whole-Grains

Whole-Wheat Flour

First, what exactly does 100% whole-wheat mean? Both whole-wheat flour and white flour come from wheat, specifically the wheat kernel. What makes commercial-made flours different is the milling process of the wheat kernel. The wheat kernel is made up of three distinct parts: the endosperm, the bran, and the germ. The endosperm contains the highest nutritional value of protein, carbohydrates, and iron, as well as trace amounts of B-complex vitamins, and is about 83% of the kernel weight. Although the bran and germ contain lower quantities of protein, they both contain larger quantities of B-complex vitamins and trace minerals, and are about 14½% and 2½% of the kernel weight, respectively. Wheat bran is the number one source of dietary fiber in wheat products.

100% whole-wheat flour contains all three parts of the kernel. Whole grains are a good source of complex carbohydrates. The wheat bran adds texture, but more importantly offers a considerable amount of dietary fiber, along with magnesium and selenium. Dietary fiber, the un-digestible carbohydrate in foods, is important to the body because it acts like a broom that sweeps out the digestive tract. The wheat germ contains polyunsaturated fat and a high amount of vitamin E, a fat-soluble vitamin and a powerful antioxidant that protects cell membranes, brain cells, and fatty molecules, such as cholesterol, from damage by free radicals. Vitamin E is important for immune system function, cancer prevention, and blood glucose control in healthy individuals, as well as in diabetics.

All-purpose (white) flour is made up of only the endosperm, which is almost all starch. During the milling process the bran and germ are removed. Enriched all-purpose flour has iron and B-vitamins added back in. But the dietary fiber is still lost and you must remember that enriched foods are never as nutritionally complete as they were in the original "whole" state. On average, one slice of whole-wheat bread contains 1.5 grams of dietary fiber, while one slice of white bread contains only 0.5 grams of dietary fiber. By removing the bran and germ during the milling process, much of the taste, texture, and approximately 80% of the nutrients are destroyed.

Oats

Oats and oatmeal are the only whole grain food that the Food and Drug Administration (FDA) recognizes as helpful in lowering cholesterol and in reducing the risk of heart disease. Because oatmeal is high in fiber, it is also helpful in maintaining healthy weight. All common forms of oats are whole grain, such as oat groats (rolled oats), old-fashioned oats, quick-cooking oats and instant oatmeal. After oats are harvested, cleaned, and roasted, they are hulled. This process does not remove the bran or the germ, so none of the fiber and none of the nutrients are lost. Not only do oats add fiber, texture, and flavor to any diet, they contain no cholesterol. Oats are high in vitamins B-1 and contain a good amount of vitamins B-2 and E.

Like wheat, oats contain the highly nutritious bran—the outer casing, which in the case of oats is high in soluble fiber. Cleanly separating the oat bran from the endosperm of the oat groats is much more difficult than separating the wheat bran from the wheat. Once removed, it is difficult to entirely separate oat bran from oat flour, so oat bran fraction will be rich in actual oat bran and contain a small amount of oat flour. While, a small amount of oat bran will remain in refined or debranned oat flour.

Stone-ground Whole Cornmeal

Corn can be eaten as both a vegetable and a grain, in the form of cornmeal. Corn kernels are composed of four distinct parts: the endosperm, germ, pericap (bran), and tip cap. Like wheat germ, the corn germ contains approximately 78% of the minerals. In the processing of corn, the germ and pericap (bran) are stripped from the endosperm. This is done to increase the shelf life of the cornmeal. Because refined cornmeal is germ-free and bran-free, much of the fiber and protein, along with B-vitamins and minerals, are lost. However, some refined cornmeal is enriched with some vitamins and minerals.

All cornmeal is milled, so you must be careful and look for "100% stone-ground whole cornmeal." The fiber, vitamin, and mineral content will be higher in whole cornmeal than in regular cornmeal. Because the pericap or bran is not removed this can limit the shelf life of the product. The pericap or bran contains two fatty acids; oleic acid and linoleic acid. Once these fatty acids oxidize they can go rancid quickly and are obviously less nutritious and can ruin the flavor of the meal. Although, fresh stone-ground whole cornmeal is always better, it is recommended that you store whole cornmeal in the refrigerator or freezer to prevent it from going rancid.

Although the majority of cornmeal is white or yellow, corn comes in a variety of colors—red, pink, black, and blue. Blue/purple corns are a more complete source of protein than either white or yellow corns. Blue cornmeal, which comes from purple corn, is quickly becoming a popular functional food. The blue/purple kernels have a sweeter nuttier taste than the white or yellow corns and the cornmeal produces a grainier coarser consistency. Although gaining in popularity as blue corn tortilla chips, blue corn flour is mostly used in making lesser-known Southwestern dishes, such as piki bread (wafer-thin cake), chaquegue (cornmeal mush), and atole (cornmeal drink). Blue/purple corn contains high amounts of anthocyanins, which are a class of plant chemicals known as flavonoids, and blue cornmeal contains higher antioxidant values than many other commercial food plants. Also, blue corn tortillas are 20% higher in protein and lower in starch than white corn tortillas.

Traditional dishes, such as white or yellow corn tortillas often include a small amount of lime, a mineral complex of calcium oxide, not the fruit. This mineral plays an important role in the body's ability to absorb niacin (vitamin B-3). The lime helps to free the niacin so that it is available for absorption. White and yellow cornmeal, prepared with lime, has been shown to prevent pellagra, a vitamin B-3 (niacin) deficiency. There are other ways to eat cornmeal: such as a polenta, which is a boiled, slow-cooked cornmeal "mush" that is made with coarsely ground yellow cornmeal and is popular in some regions of Italy; and hominy grits from which corn grits are made.

Rye

Rye is another good grain to include in your diet. This grain is commonly used to make both rye and pumpernickel breads. Rye grain is longer and more slender than wheat and is available in whole or cracked grain form. Because it is difficult to separate the bran and germ from the endosperm, many of the nutrients in refined rye flour are not lost. This makes rye flour better than wheat flour, in most cases. Although, one drawback is that the gluten in rye flour is less elastic and therefore breads made from rye flour will have a tendency to be more compact and dense. Rye is a good source of fiber and has a high water-binding capacity, which gives you a feeling of being full. More nutrients and fiber are retained in refined rye flour than in refined wheat flour. Because rye bread is more compact and dense, the rate at which starchs (carbohydrates) are broken down and metabolized into sugar is much slower than with wheat flour.

Barley

Barley is a cereal grain that in most forms does not lose it nutritional value once it has been processed. Barley is found in many forms. Hulled barley, with its indigestible outer hull of the barley removed, still has the whole bran. Pot/scotch barley, although processed, still contains a portion of the bran. Barley flakes, which are flattened and sliced and appear similar to rolled oats. Barley grits, which is barley that has been toasted and cracked, appears similar to bulgar. Pearl barley has the fiber-rich bran removed through the milling process. Because most forms of barley are high in dietary fiber, they provide the bulk your intestines need and decrease the time it takes for fecal matter to be expelled from the body. The dietary fiber in barley is high in beta glucan, which helps to lower cholesterol by binding to the bile acids and removing them rapidly from the body.

Although, there numerous other grains that I did not cover that may be your favorite, it is important that you do your own research to see how they are milled and processed, what nutrients and minerals are retained and lost, what the nutritional values are for the refined product, and most importantly if you can purchase them in a 100% whole grain state.

Rice and Other Grains

Wild Rice

Wild rice is actually not rice, but is a seed in the family of grasses. It is native to North America and grows "wild" predominately in the Great Lakes area, although it has been "cultivated" and adapted in some states, such as California and Idaho. Native Americans called it *Manomin* or "good berry." Early European settlers referred to wild rice as Indian rice, water oats, and marsh oats. This rice is almost always sold as a whole grain. Wild rice is richer in protein than white rice and most other grains, and contains more niacin than brown rice.

It is high in complex carbohydrates and contains lysine—an amino acid that is found in very few grains. It is also low in sodium and is a good source of fiber, calcium, B-vitamins, and minerals. Because of all the nutritional value wild rice offers, it has become very popular among health-food enthusiasts and consumers in general. You can easily find rice blends that include wild rice. This is convenient because this allows you to try these blends and adjust to the flavor and texture of wild rice.

This rice has a distinctive texture and flavor and is an excellent substitute for potatoes or white rice, especially alongside fish. It can also be used in a variety of dishes, such as wild rice stuffing/dressing and soups. Some people find the taste of wild rice too strong and even bitter. This may be because it has not been properly rinsed before preparation. The secret to preparing perfect wild rice is simple: make sure that you rinse the rice thoroughly (this may require that you rinse multiple times with cold water) before cooking, until the water looks clear.

Brown Rice

Brown rice is really white rice that hasn't been milled and polished. In order to fully comprehend what this means, we need to look at the process of refining rice. A grain of whole rice, in its natural state, is composed of several layers. In order to be able to eat brown rice, the outer layer or hull must be removed. Since the hull does not contain any nutritional value, removing it only makes the rice edible. Removing most of the germ layer and all of the bran from brown rice makes the rice appear whiter, and with far less nutrients. In order to get even whiter rice and to extend the shelf life of the product, the rice is then polished, a process in which the aleurone layer, which is the innermost layer of the grain of the rice, is removed. What is left is only a refined starch that has little nutritional value. Much of the nutritional value of rice is destroyed through the milling and polishing process. In total, 67% of the vitamin B-3, 80% of the vitamin B-1, 90% of the vitamin B-6, half of the manganese and phosphorous, 60% of the iron, and all of the dietary fiber and essential fatty acids are lost. Although white rice is enriched, it is only enriched with vitamins B-1, B-3, and niacin and 11 of the lost nutrients are not replaced in any form. Because it is less processed, brown rice contains four times the amount of insoluble fiber of white rice. Also, it has more texture and flavor than white rice. However, because it is a whole grain, the cooking time will be slightly longer. It can be used as a substitute for potatoes or white rice, and it is especially flavorful and complementary in Asian dishes.

Specialty Rice

Exotic colored rice, such as the Himalayan and Bhutanese Red, the Forbidden Chinese Black, and the Green Bamboo are also available. Because of their stunning colors, and their lighter, sweeter texture and flavor, they are gaining popularity. Some of these types of rice can be used in desserts or simply steamed and served along with fruits, such as mango. As with any rice, you need to be careful, and remember that all rice is not created equal. Some colored rice are milled or partially milled, while others are considered whole grain. The nutritional value of each type of rice will depend on how the rice was processed. So, it is important to ensure you purchase 100% whole grain rice.

Himalayan and Bhutanese Red rice is grown in the foothills of the Himalayas in the small Asian nation of Bhutan. This rice has a thin bran coating, which can be partially milled. This red rice has the same nutritional value as brown rice, but because of its thin bran coating cooks in almost half the time. Black Chinese rice is not milled, so its purple-black bran layer is left intact on the grain. This iron-rich black rice is also known as Forbidden rice or Emperor's rice. In ancient times this rice was served only to the emperor to preserve his health and longevity. This particular rice has a roasted nutty flavor, with a hint of citrus. Green Bamboo rice is actually short grain white rice that has been infused with the chlorophyll from pure bamboo juice. The chlorophyll gives this white rice its stunning green color and unique flavor. When cooked, Bamboo rice will have a mild green tea flavor with a sticky quality similar to sushi rice.

An American-grown rice that is slowly regaining its popularity is the Carolina Gold, which has a light, buttery taste. Originally from Madagascar, the Carolina Gold is now grown on southeast rice plantations from North Carolina to northern Florida. Although this rice is actually white in color, it gets its name from the "golden" color of the tall rice stalks in the field. Unfortunately, this rice is very fragile, and can be broken easily during the milling process when the bran is removed. As with any rice that is milled, most of the Carolina Gold's nutritional value is lost.

Quinoa

Quinoa (pronounced keen—wah), a rediscovered ancient "grain," also known as "the gold of the Incas" and "the mother grain," is quickly becoming known as one of the best "supergrains" of today. Just as wild rice that is related to grasses is not a true grain, quinoa, also is not an actual grain, but is instead the seed of a green leafy plant that is related to spinach and Swiss chard. The most typical color of quinoa is a transparent yellow grain, although it can be found in a variety of colors—orange, pink, red, purple, or black. Quinoa is an excellent complete protein, because it is one of the few grains that contain lysine—an amino acid that is essential for tissue growth and repair. As a complete protein, it contains all nine essential amino acids. It also is a good source of B-vitamins and minerals. Although it is low in gluten, quinoa flour can be combined with wheat flour in making baked goods and can also be used to make pasta. When preparing quinoa, make sure that you rinse it thoroughly, as with wild rice, to ensure that any remaining saponin, the bitter soapy coating, is removed. Quinoa is prepared the same as white rice, with the water to quinoa ratio of 2:1. Cooked quinoa is translucent with the germ spiraled out from the grain. When cooked, it has a fluffy and creamy, but slightly crunchy texture with a nutty to neutral flavor.

Teff

Teff is another one of the fastest growing "supergrains" on the market and one of the most nutrient-dense grains. The most typical color of teff is a khaki-colored grain which closely resembles millet. Although, there are three main colors; white, red, and brown, the colors within each category can vary widely from ivory to light tan to deep brown or dark-reddish purple. This whole grain is believed to have originated in Ethiopia between 4000 and 1000 B.C. The name teff is derived from the Amharic word "teffa," which means "lost." This refers to how easily this tiny grain is lost when harvested as it drops to the ground. It is the smallest grain in the world, measuring only 1/32 of an inch in diameter, and it would take 150 teff grains to be equal in weight to one wheat grain. Because of its small size, it is almost entirely made up of bran and germ, the most nutritious part of any grain. Teff is a nutrient dense grain, which is very high in calcium, phosphorous, iron, copper, aluminum, barium, and thiamin; as well as being high in protein, carbohydrates, and fiber. Just like quinoa, teff has higher lysine levels than wheat or barley. One of the main advantages of this grain is that it is gluten free, so that persons who are gluten intolerant or have Celiac disease have a viable option in this whole grain. This particular grain is very versatile and can be used as a side, along any meat, poultry, or fish, or as a hot cereal, may be added to soups and stews, and added to flour in baking. Teff is prepared in a similar way as quinoa. When preparing teff as a hot cereal, the water to teff ratio is 4:1. When cooked, it has a creamy texture with a mild, nutty, and a slightly molasses sweetness.

Chia

Another ancient "supergrain" that is quickly gaining popularity is the Chia seed, which is better known as the novelty gift, the Chia pet which grows its own "hair." Chia seeds come from a plant in the mint family known as Salvia Hispanica. In pre-Columbian times, the plant Salvia Hispanica was a component of Aztec and Mayan diets and Chia was a major crop in central and southern Mexico. The seeds were used by the Indigenous peoples of the region in religious ceremonies. In the 16th century, after the Spanish conquest, it was banned because of its association with the Aztec "pagan" religion. The "hair" of this plant is actually similar to alfalfa sprouts and can be used in much the same way. This seed which is edible, is higher in omega-3 fatty acids than flaxseed but, unlike flaxseeds, can be stored for long periods of time without going rancid and do not require grinding for consumption. According to a team of researchers from St. Michael's Hospital in Toronto, 3.5 ounces of Chia seeds contain the same amount of omega-3 fatty acids as 28 ounces of salmon, as much calcium as three cups of milk, and as much iron as five cups of raw spinach. Chia seeds contain high levels of fiber, calcium, magnesium, omega-3 fatty acids, and more anti-oxidants than many berries. The Chia seed, which is either white or black, has a slightly nutty flavor and is gluten-free. The seeds can be eaten whole as a snack, or when ground can be sprinkled on hot or cold cereals, yogurt, or salads and can be added to any flour when making baked goods.

The water-soluble fiber, in oats and barley, helps the intestines to bind and eliminate cholesterol from your body and therefore may provide extra heart protection. The FDA stated that women need at least 25g of fiber daily for maximum heart protection. According to a recent study of 10,000 people, women at the high end of the scale averaged 21g of fiber per day and those at the lowest averaged 6g. The same study found that with a diet high in fiber, the risk of developing heart disease was lowered up to 15% (*Prevention*, May 2004, p. 80).

A Harvard study found 49% of those who ate 2 or more servings of whole grains, in foods, such as bread, cereal, and rice, were less likely to be overweight. Whole grains burn more calories during digestion, help you feel full longer, and trigger lower fat-storing insulin than refined carbohydrates (*Prevention*, June 2004, p. 64).

Whole grains are better than refined grains. The germ of whole wheat provides vitamin E, thiamin, folic acid, phosphorus, magnesium, zinc, and iron, while the bran is loaded with fiber, which fills you up without adding calories. Overweight people who were given low-fat, high-fiber meals over a three-month period lost an average of seven pounds without even trying (*Natural Health*: Special Issue, Summer 2005, p. 58).

Milk, Yogurt, & Cheese (Dairy)

Of the many sources of calcium, dairy foods are among the highest. Calcium is required in several key processes; it is necessary for the body to build strong teeth and bones, build bone mass, and maintain bone density to help prevent osteoporosis. Calcium is also necessary for the proper function of the heart, muscles, and nervous system. Dairy foods contain protein, and when combined with vegetable protein it increases the nutritional value of the vegetable protein. Dairy foods are also an excellent source of B vitamins, such as riboflavin. Most dairy products now contain vitamin D, which helps the body absorb the calcium, as well as other important minerals, such as selenium, zinc, phosphorus, potassium, and magnesium. Some dairy products may contain probiotics, which are simply "good" bacteria. Probiotic bacteria, used to make cultured dairy products, such as yogurt, help your body maintain a good balance of bacteria in your intestinal tract and may help protect against cancer and high cholesterol.

Recommended USDA daily requirements (based on a 2,000 calorie diet):

❖ Milk products provide protein, vitamins, and minerals. Milk, yogurt, and cheese are the best source of calcium. Choose skim milk and nonfat yogurt.

❖ Eat 2 to 3 servings each day: 2 servings for most people, and 3 servings for women who are pregnant or breastfeeding, teenagers, and young adults to age 24.

Examples of serving sizes:

> ➢ 1 cup of skim milk or nonfat yogurt
> ➢ 1 ½ ounces of natural cheese
> ➢ 2 ounces of processed cheese

Milk

Milk, specifically cow's milk, is the basis of most dairy products on the market. Milk is considered a nearly complete food and a nutrient dense food. In relation to the small amount of calories milk provides a high amount of vitamins and minerals per serving. Not only is milk an excellent source of calcium, it also provides eight essential nutrients—vitamins A, B-12, and D (when vitamin D fortified), riboflavin (a B vitamin), phosphorus, potassium, niacin, and protein. An eight-ounce serving of vitamin D fortified milk provides 30% of the daily value of calcium, 25% of the daily value for vitamins B and D, 23% of the daily value for phosphorus, 39% of the daily value of iodine, and 16.3% of the daily value for protein.

Like meats and poultry, milk is graded and compliance to the grading process is voluntary. Milk that is Grade A must be pasteurized. Pasteurized milk is heated to destroy the disease-causing bacteria, yeast, and mold in milk. This process also increases the shelf life of milk, but does not destroy the nutritional values. It is estimated that 99% of all milk in the markets is pasteurized according to the standards set by the FDA and the United States Public Health Service. Homogenized milk ensures that the milkfat is evenly distributed in the milk by forcing the milk through a small opening at a high pressure. This process helps to break down the fat particles and prevents them from separating. Although the pasteurization and homogenization processes are voluntary, they make milk healthier and easier to consume.

Milk comes in many forms—whole milk, reduced fat or 2% milk, low-fat or 1% milk, and skim or fat free milk. Whole milk must contain at least 3.5% of milkfat and 8.25% milk solids by weight and gets approximately 50% of its calories from fat; reduced fat milk contains 2% milkfat and gets approximately 35% of its calories from fat; low-fat contains 1% milkfat and gets approximately 23% of its calories for fat; while skim or fat-free cannot contain more than 0.5% milkfat and gets approximately 5% of its calories from fat. Also, no matter which type of milk you consume, each contains approximately the same amount of lactose or milk sugar.

All basic non-evaporated varieties of milk provide the same amount of calcium and the eight essential nutrients. For example, eight ounces of whole milk contains 8 grams of fat, 150 calories, and 13 grams of sugar, reduced fat or 2% milk contains 5 grams of fat, 120 calories, and 13 grams of sugar, low-fat or 1% milk contains 2.5 grams of fat, 100 calories, and 12 grams of sugar, and skim or fat free milk contains no fat, 80 calories, and 12 grams of sugar, while all four contain 300 mg of calcium. Many people are concerned that whole milk and whole milk products are both higher in calories and fat and so the trend of consuming the lower fat milk and milk products is gaining popularity and consuming these products is generally a good change to make in your diet.

There are also specialty milks, such as buttermilk, lactose-reduced milk, and low-sodium milk to name a few, and various dry and canned milks, such as evaporated and sweetened and unsweetened condensed. Old-fashioned homemade buttermilk is not a buttery, high-fat milk, but is actually the slightly sour, residual liquid which remains after butter is churned. So, buttermilk is the milk from the butter. Buttermilks will have a slightly sour taste, which is similar in taste to yogurt, and have a slightly thicker texture than regular cow's milk, but thinner than heavy cream. On average, it takes about one gallon of milk to yield ½ pint of true old-fashioned homemade buttermilk. Most commercial buttermilk is made by adding a lactic acid bacteria culture to any pasteurized sweet milk, either the whole or fat-free (skim) milks. This mixture is left to ferment for approximately 12-14 hours at a low temperature. Commercial buttermilk is usually labeled "cultured buttermilk," may contain added salt, and is lower in fat than sweet milk.

Although, milk is recommended as part of a healthy nutritional diet, one needs to understand which type of milk is best for each individual. Whole milk should be consumed by infants and children, two years old and under. Reduced fat or 2% milk is a good milk to choose for those consuming lower amounts of fat in their diet. Because reduced fat milk is still high in fat, it should be used to transition you from whole milk to low-fat or 1% milk. Low-fat or 1% milk is a good compromise to make in one's diet. This offers the calcium and other essential nutrients, along with the lower calorie and fat content. Skim or fat free milk is also a good choice for most adults and those on very strict low-fat diets. Although many dieters find this milk to be too "thin" and the light bluish tinge is considered by many to be unappealing.

If you have a lactose-intolerance or just do not like the flavor of cow's milk, then you may want to try non-dairy milks. Many stores are now selling many different types of non-dairy milks, such as soymilk, nut milks, and grain milks. The important nutritional information about these non-dairy products is that they are plant-based, they contain no cholesterol and, in many cases, contain little to no saturated fats. Each type of plant-based milk has its own distinct texture, color, and taste. Also, not all non-dairy milks are fortified with calcium and vitamin D, so it is important that you read the label to ensure that you are purchasing one that is fortified.

Soymilk, the most popular non-dairy milk, contains soy protein and isoflavones which have been shown to modestly decrease "bad" LDL cholesterol levels. However, soymilk does have slightly less protein than cow's milk and unfortified soymilk contains little absorbable calcium. Nut milks, such as almond, hazelnut, and Brazil nut, are quickly gaining popularity. Nut milks are made from ground nuts that have been strained, liquefied, and then sweetened to balance the slightly bitter taste. Because some nut milks are sweetened with refined cane sugars or juices, it is recommended that you purchase the unsweetened varieties. Also nut milks have less protein than soymilks and most are not fortified with vitamins and minerals. Lastly, there are the grain milks, such as rice and oats. Because these milks are made from grains, which have natural fiber present, they will have the added benefit of fiber naturally infused into the drink. Like nut milks, grain milks will contain less protein and may be sweetened with refined cane sugar or juice. So it is recommended that you purchase the unsweetened varieties.

Lastly, there are two other non-dairy milks that are becoming more recognized and going mainstream: coconut milk and hemp milk. Coconut milk is made from the meat of the coconut, not the liquid that is drained from the coconut once it has been punctured. The flesh or meat is found along the inner walls of the coconut, which is finely grated and steeped in hot water. Next the pieces are squeezed through cheesecloth and this liquid collected is the coconut milk. Coconut milk can have various consistencies, from thick and creamy to thin and lighter. Although high in saturated fat, it is the much healthier plant-based saturated fats—capric and lauric acid, which support the body's immune system. Lauric acid, which is also found in mother's milk, has been shown to promote brain development and bone health. Coconut milk also contains anti-carcinogenic, anti-microbial, anti-bacterial, and anti-viral qualities. Like other non-dairy milks, coconut milk comes in sweetened and unsweetened forms and in a variety of flavors, such as vanilla.

Hemp milk is made from the "nuts" or seeds of the industrial hemp plant. Because this plant is illegal for U.S. farmers to grow, a number of hemp milks producers use the seeds from Canada where hemp grows legally. Although the seeds and fibers contain only trace amounts of the psychoactive tetrahydrocannabinol (THC), hemp milk is THC-free. Hemp milk is touted as a balanced source of omega-3 and omega-6 fatty acids, a quality protein, is calcium and iron rich, and is fortified with other vitamins and minerals, including D2, B12, and riboflavin. Hemp milk does not contain dairy, tree nuts, soy, cholesterol, or cane sugar, and like other non-dairy alternative comes in a variety of flavors, such as vanilla and chocolate.

Yogurt

For more than 30 years, yogurt has been a favorite among health food enthusiasts, and with good reason. Yogurt is not only a quick and easy snack, but it is nutritious, as well. While yogurt is a healthy snack, it is not a healthy meal. Many people have opted to replace meals, especially breakfast or lunch, with a cup or two of yogurt. This is not a healthy and balanced food choice. Yogurt is a good source of calcium, vitamins and minerals. Among them are phosphorus, riboflavin (vitamin B-2), iodine, vitamin B-12, pantothenic acid (vitamin B-5), zinc, and potassium. Yogurt is also a good source of protein and molybdenum. Yogurt is also a healthy choice because it contains one thing that other dairy products do not—healthy live active bacteria.

During the culturing process of making yogurt, pasteurized and homogenized milk is inoculated with two special bacterial cultures—lactobacillus bulgaricus and streptococcus thermophilus. These two bacteria cause the lactose or milk sugar to turn into a lactic acid. This process also allows for the liquid to thicken and creates its slightly tart taste. These cultures may not only help to protect and fortify your immune system, but also enhance your immune response. The process of making yogurt creates lactase, an enzyme in which lactose intolerant people are deficient. Although the amount of lactose that remains in yogurt may fluctuate from 25% to 80%, the presence of lactase means eating yogurt may still be a better way for those who are lactose intolerant to get their recommended daily allowance of dairy. The live cultures may also help with the digestion of milk protein, restore and balance the "good" bacteria in the intestines, and may kill the "bad" bacteria, such as listeria and salmonella.

Some yogurts, such as Swiss-style, or frozen yogurts are pasteurized a second time, which then destroys the live active bacteria. This second pasteurization is also known as "heat-treated after culturing." To ensure that you get the healthiest benefit from consuming yogurt, make sure that the label clearly states the presence of the "live bacteria cultures."

Yogurt comes in many varieties—skim or fat free, low-fat, and regular or whole milk. Obviously there is no fat in the fat free yogurt, which is an excellent choice for those attempting to limit fat in their diets. However, in some yogurts there may be added or hidden sugars, which can offset the reduction of fat with higher calories. An eight-ounce serving of low-fat yogurt contains approximately two to five grams of fat, while eight ounces of regular yogurt contains approximately six to eight grams of fat.

There are four types of yogurt, plain or unflavored, flavored, and two types of yogurt with fruit already added—sundae-style and Swiss- or French-style. Plain yogurt is the most versatile because you can eat it plain, add fresh fruit if you choose, or use it as a base for other dishes, such as a chip dip or a cucumber sauce. An eight-ounce cup is approximately 110 to 140 calories. Flavored yogurt, with contains no fruit solids, sundae-style yogurt, which contains fruit on the bottom that must be mixed and blended, and Swiss- or French-style yogurt, which contains fruit pre-mixed in the yogurt, are approximately 100 to 307 calories per eight-ounce serving. Also, for those who are lactose-intolerant, there is a growing alternative trend in non-dairy yogurt, such soy-based and coconut-based yogurts. The key to making sure yogurt remains a healthier choice, is to ensure that no added or hidden sugars are in the product. The addition of processed sugars, especially high fructose corn syrup, will add to the total calories consumed and in some cases can make yogurt a less than healthy choice.

Cheese

Cheese and cheese products come in many varieties—with more than 300 varieties produced and sold in the United States and more than 1,400 varieties of cheese worldwide. Cheese is a good source of calcium, as well as vitamins and minerals. Cheese is considered a high-quality protein because it contains a good complement of essential amino acids in proportion to our body's needs. All cheeses are a good nutrient dense food. For example, a one-ounce serving of part-skim mozzarella cheese provides 18.3% of the daily value of calcium, 13% of the daily value for phosphorus, 6.7% of the daily value of iodine, 5.8% of selenium, and 13.8% of the daily value for protein, while only 72 calories.

The milk that is used to make cheese can come from several sources—cow, sheep, or goat. Cheese and cheese products are determined by the type of milk used, how they are processed, and what the tastes, preferences, and the cooking needs are for the consumer. It takes approximately 5 quarts of whole milk to make 1 pound of whole milk cheese. As with all types of milk, all types of cheese will provide a good source of calcium, vitamins, and minerals. The type of milk that is used will determine the taste and texture of the cheese. Cheese is made with whole milk, reduced or 2% milk, low-fat or 1% milk, skim or fat free milk, or a combination of these milks. Regardless of which type you choose from, it is recommended that you choose a low-fat or part-skim cheese. You will still get the nutritional benefits, such as calcium, but also avoid the higher fat and calorie content in whole milk cheeses.

There are several ways to classify cheeses—natural, processed, and cheese powders. Natural cheeses are generally made from pasteurized milk. There are several categories of natural cheese, which are categorized by their level of softness or hardness: soft cheeses, which include Brie, ricotta, cottage cheese; semi-soft cheeses, which include blue, brick, feta, mozzarella, Monterey Jack; hard cheeses, which include cheddar, Colby, gouda, Swiss; and very hard cheeses, which include parmesan and Romano, to name a few. Processed cheeses are a blending of one or more natural cheeses but contain more moisture than natural cheeses. Processed cheeses include American cheese, cheese spreads, and cheese foods. Cheese powders are dehydrated cheeses that can be made from pure cheese or a blend of cheeses, food ingredients, and food color. These are usually found in dry mixes, sauces, and snack foods. Aged cheeses, which contain little to no lactose, are especially good for those people that are lactose intolerant. As in non-dairy milk and yogurt alternatives, there are numerous non-dairy cheeses available, such as goat cheese, soy cheese, and a wide variety of nut cheeses.

Researchers found that drinking one glass of milk daily could reduce the risk for developing colon cancer, the third most common cancer among women. Subjects who drank at least 8.5 ounces of milk daily were 15% less likely to get colon cancer than those who drank almost none. Also, the fatty acids found in milk may help to reduce the levels of the most artery-damaging forms of cholesterol (*Natural Health*: Special Issue, Summer 2005, p. 15).

Fat-free half & half, sour cream, and cream cheese could reduce your caloric intake by several hundred calories a day. For example, 2 tablespoons of fat-free half & half is 20 calories and 3 grams of fat less than 2 tablespoons of cream. Over a one-year period, that can equal a 2-pound weight loss (*Natural Health*: Special Issue, Summer 2005, p. 23).

The "good" bacteria in yogurt, such as lactobacillus bulgaricus or acidophilus, streptococcus thermophilus, and bifidobacterium, increase the absorption of nutrients, reduce the symptoms of lactose intolerance, and may fight cancer. These bacteria live in the intestinal tract, where they crowd out disease-causing bacteria, and possibly turn off an enzyme that triggers colon cancer. Yogurts should contain LAC (live active culture) that list acidophilus and bifidobacterium as ingredients. Also, yogurt is a great source of calcium. But choose plain non-fat varieties, since most commercial fruited yogurt can contain as much as 9 teaspoons of added sugar (*Natural Health*: Special Issue, Summer 2005, p. 25).

If you are lactose intolerant, yogurt is the easiest dairy food to digest. A new study found that yogurt works as well as milk and cheese for losing weight. Eighteen women who ate 500 fewer calories and 6 ounces of yogurt three times a day for 12 weeks lost 3.6 more pounds and 1.2 more inches from their waists than 16 women who also cut calories but ate no yogurt (*Prevention*, August 2005, p. 75).

Fats, Oils, & Sweets

As I stated earlier, this can be the most difficult of the food groups to understand because many foods contain fats. Not all fats are oils, but all oils are fats. Fats, especially saturated fats, are found in animal and animal-based products. Because details on saturated fats were already included within other sections of this book related to certain foods, such as meats, nuts, and milk, I will concentrate on the cooking fats and oils that are used to prepare foods, not the fats that are contained within a particular food or food group. Also, many sweets and pastries are very high in saturated fats, such as butter, margarine, shortening, and (partially) hydrogenated oils, also known as trans fats, which are even worse than saturated fats.

Fats and Oils

The majority of commercial oils are plant-based. All plant-based oils are liquid fat and contain no cholesterol. Only animal-based foods contain cholesterol. The right types of oils are important to our diet because they not only are a good source of energy, but they supply our body with essential fatty acids, which are the building blocks of cell membranes. These fatty acids help the body to absorb many of the vitamins found in the foods we consume, including vitamins A, D, E, and K. Also, fatty acids contribute to healthier skin. Although, these essential fatty acids may be beneficial, the oils they are found in are very high in calories. One tablespoon of any oil is about 120 calories and approximately 14 grams of fat. The amount of saturated fat will vary depending on the type of oil used. "Light" oil refers only to the flavor and taste of the oil and has nothing to do with the calories or fat per serving.

Recommended USDA daily requirements (based on a 2,000 calorie diet):

❖   Consume these sparingly.

Everyone has heard about eliminating the "hidden" fats, limiting the "wrong" fats, and adding the "right" fats in any diet. First, let's begin by breaking down these oils or fats into their three types and second, looking at the qualities of these types of cooking oils. There are three types of fats: saturated fats, monounsaturated fats, and polyunsaturated fats. All vegetable oils contain a mixture of these three fats. Saturated fats are found predominately in animal products and in some vegetables and are solid at room temperature. Saturated fats contain long chain, medium chain, and short chain fats. Long chain fats are shown to raise blood cholesterol. There are studies that indicate a diet high in saturated fats may lead to higher risks of cardiovascular disease and other chronic illnesses, such as diabetes. This is the "bad" or "wrong" fat that you need to limit, but not eliminate, in your diet.

The healthier "good" fats are the unsaturated fats: monounsaturated and polyunsaturated. Monounsaturated fats remain liquid at room temperature, but once refrigerated will become cloudy and thick. This fat contains the Omega-9 (oleic acid) fatty acid, which is the main fatty acid found in olive oil. Oleic acid has been shown to decrease "bad" LDL cholesterol, while leaving the "good" HDL cholesterol alone. This fatty acid also has a beneficial effect on heart health, other chronic illnesses, and certain cancers. The olive tree is a major source of oleic acid, but canola and chocolate are also good sources. Monounsaturated fats can be found in their highest concentration in canola oil, olive oils, safflower and sunflower oils, and peanut, hazelnut, and macadamia nut oils.

Polyunsaturated fats will remain liquid at room temperature and in the refrigerator. This fat contains two classes of fatty acids: Omega-3 (linolenic acid) and Omega-6 (linoleic acid). Because the body cannot produce these two fatty acids and they can only be added through diet, they are considered essential fatty acids. So it is important to include polyunsaturated fats in your diet. The most common recommendation of Omega-3 to Omega-6 ratio is a 2:1 daily intake. Omega-3 fatty acids have been shown to decrease blood cholesterol, have anti-inflammatory properties, and may prevent some types of chronic illnesses. Omega-3 fatty acids can be found in their highest concentration in flaxseed oil, walnut oil, and canola oils, while Omega-6 fatty acids can be found in at higher concentrations in corn and soybean oils.

A fourth type of fat is what I call the "hidden fat" — (partially) hydrogenated oils or trans fatty acids/trans fats. Trans fats are a man-made "bad" fat that is made by converting unsaturated "good" fat into a saturated "bad" fat. Trans fats are known as (partially) hydrogenated oil and any type of oil can be made into a trans fat. Whenever a product uses any kind (partially) hydrogenated oils, trans fatty acids will be present in the final product. There is increasing evidence that trans fats may increase total blood cholesterol and the "bad" LDL cholesterol more than regular saturated fats. Also, trans fats can interfere with the way your body produces and uses the "good" HDL cholesterol. Therefore, you should avoid products that contain trans fats and/or (partially) hydrogenated vegetable oils. Although monounsaturated and polyunsaturated fats are considered healthy fats, they can break down and become unhealthy trans fats. When overheated, these unsaturated fats have at least one unsaturated bond that can become hydrogenated or saturated. When purchasing oils, make sure the label states that the oil was "cold-pressed" and that you discard the oil once it has been used or heated to its smoke point.

You need to understand that you cannot use only one type of oil, such as canola oil, for all types of cooking. So it is recommended that you understand which oil is better for the type of cooking or use. Different oils have different smoke points, which simply is the point to which the oil can be heated without smoking. If any oil burns beyond the smoke point, then hydrogenation will occur, which means a trans fat will be produced. Oils that are good for baking may be bad for frying. For example, flaxseed oil has an extremely low smoke point and should never be used to cook foods. Butter and margarine also have a low smoke point, so you can use them to sauté, but not fry foods. Olive oil has a medium smoke point and it is best used as a salad dressing or for baking and to lightly sauté. Refined sunflower oil has a higher smoke point so you can easily use it to sauté and fry foods, but not for deep frying foods. Although canola oil has a higher smoke point than most other oils and can be used for deep frying, peanut oil has one of the highest smoke points and is, therefore, an even better choice for deep frying foods.

As with any food, I use the same criteria when choosing cooking oils; I try to pick the oils that are lower in saturated fats, higher in monounsaturated and polyunsaturated fats, and choose products that do not contain (partially) hydrogenated oils or trans fatty acids. Because there are numerous "good" oils to choose from, I will highlight some of the more commonly used oils. The following charts will highlight and compare the percentages (to 100%) of saturated, monounsaturated, and polyunsaturated fats in these common oils and fats and their smoke point (if applicable). The charts will list them from lowest to highest in saturated fat.

Oils:	Saturated	Monounsaturated	Polyunsaturated	Smoke Point (By degrees)
Canola oil	7	58	35	400
Flaxseed oil	9	19	72	225
Grapeseed oil	9	14	77	400
Safflower oil	9	13	78	450
Sunflower oil	11	20	69	450
Corn oil	13	25	62	400
Olive oil	14	74	12	350
Walnut oil	14	19	67	400
Sesame oil	15	42	43	400
Soybean oil	15	24	61	450
Peanut oil	18	49	33	450
Rice bran oil	20	47	33	490
Palm oil	52	38	10	350
Coconut oil	92	6	2	375

Fats:	Saturated	Monounsaturated	Polyunsaturated
Margarine, tub *	17	46	37
Margarine, whipped *	20	50	30
Lard	41	47	12
Cocoa butter	62	35	3
Butter	66	30	4
Butterfat	68	28	4
Butter, whipped	69	28	3

* use trans fat free varieties only

Although, coconut oil, which is extremely high in saturated fat, has gotten a bad reputation, some studies are now indicating that it may actually be a healthy oil to add to your diet. Coconut oil is a natural plant-based saturated fat, not an animal saturated fat or a man-made trans fat. Recent studies also show that oils higher in saturated fats, such as coconut oil, are more stable when heated than the unsaturated oils and cannot be damaged by higher heating temperatures. It is also made up of short and medium chain triglycerides (SCTs and MCTs). There is growing evidence that MCTs may encourage muscle tissue growth and repair. Because MCTs are absorbed directly into the liver, this makes them more readily available for energy. Also MCTs promote satiety, which is the feeling of being full, thus deceasing hunger and helping to control weight.

How you will be using the oil, to either sauté, fry, stir-fry, or deep fry, will determine which types of oil you could choose from. Also, different oils have different flavors and will have a different effect on how the final food will taste. The taste of oils will vary from bland, to neutral, to mild, to mildly nutty, to nutty. Choosing the oil to use in your kitchen will depend on your personal tastes and how you want to incorporate the oil into a meal. For example, I use canola oil for baking and stir-frying; olive oil to make salad dressings and in my pizza crust, organic all vegetable shortening in my bread dough, and canola, peanut or grapeseed oil to deep fry. I have also tried corn, almond, and walnut oil, on occasion. Sometimes it is nice to try other oils and see how they change the flavor of your recipes.

Sweets

If you have at least tried to change your old eating habits by consuming foods according to the recommended daily allowance from the food groups detailed above, and by trying to incorporate my four basic rules, then you should be well on your way to eliminating the higher saturated fats, white flour, sweets, and pastries from your diet. By simply eating more naturally sweet fruits and by preparing and serving them in more creative ways, you can slowly reduce your cravings for unhealthy desserts and pastries. Because of the amount of "bad" saturated fats, trans fats, processed sugars, and white flour used to prepare the majority of cakes, pies, cookies, etc., it is important that you reduce commercially prepared sweets as much as possible. What you need to focus on is how to modify the types of sweets you and your family enjoy. Although, you do not need to entirely eliminate all sweets from your diet, you should, in moderation, always try to eat healthy sweets that contain unrefined flour, natural unrefined sugars, and "good" fats.

Therefore, the key for this category is to become more aware of which types of sweets and pastry products are healthier. For example, dark chocolate is quickly gaining legitimacy from various researchers as a heart-healthy food. Although, this does not give you license to eat a slice of double chocolate cake every day. Chocolate comes from cocoa beans, which contains a substantial amount of natural antioxidants or polyphenols, specifically flavonoids. Studies are showing that two specific types of flavonols—catechins and procyanidins—can have positive health effects. First, these antioxidants are instrumental in preventing free radical damage, by preventing arterial damage. Free radical damage can lead to heart disease and other chronic diseases related to aging. Second, they may also play a role in lowering the risk of heart attack or stroke by inhibiting the growth of clots in blood vessels. Chocolate also contains serotonin, which acts as an anti-depressant, along with a number of healthy nutrients. It is high in potassium and magnesium and provides the body with vitamins, including B1, B2, and E.

Although dark chocolate, ounce for ounce, contains approximately five times as many antioxidants as blueberries, it is a calorie-dense food, meaning it is much higher in calories, especially when compared to other healthy nutrient-dense foods. An ounce of dark chocolate, depending on type and brand, can have approximately 100 to 200 calories. Also, chocolate contains saturated and unsaturated fats. There are several ways to incorporate chocolate, especially dark chocolate, into your diet while keeping it a healthy choice. First, this is one area that I would stress: buy only organic or name brands, to avoid unhealthy additives, such as (high) fructose corn syrup and (partially) hydrogenated oils, and to ensure that it has pure minimally processed sugars, such as (evaporated) cane juice. Second, you should always buy chocolate products that are at least 70% cocoa, because the higher the cocoa content the more antioxidants it will contain. Lastly, you should also choose to buy natural minimally sweetened, unsweetened, or sugar-free dark chocolates, but remember that unsweetened and sugar-free is not calorie-free. All researchers stress that consuming any chocolate product in moderation is the key.

Recommended UMIM* recommended serving per week:

❖   Up to 7 ounces per week, average 1 ounce per day.
    * The University of Michigan Integrative Medicine Clinical Services (UMIM) developed their own Healing Food Pyramid and the recommendations listed above can be found on the UMIM: Healing Food Pyramid Internet website - http:www. med.umich.edu/umim/clinical/pyramid. This website also provides detailed information on other foods within the major food groups.

There are many healthy ways to incorporate a little bit of cocoa and chocolate into your diet. First, you must know which type to choose in order to incorporate them in the desserts and pastries you will eat. In order to make chocolate products, roasted and fermented cocoa beans are crushed into a liquid. This chocolate liquor is then used to make various chocolate products. Let's begin by looking at a few of the many different types of cocoa products available to include into your diet plan.

The fat in chocolate liquor is removed and the chocolate solids that remain are ground up to become cocoa powder. Because cocoa powder is the least processed, it contains the highest amount of flavonoids. It also does not contain any added sugars, and therefore, is the healthiest of the cocoa products. Because it has no sugar, it will have a bitter taste. The best way to incorporate this into your diet is by adding it to other dishes. For example, add it to the batters for sweeter breads, like banana or zucchini, or add it to hot milk for hot chocolate.

Baking chocolate is basically chocolate liquor that has cooled and hardened. It will contain the cocoa butter, so it will be higher in fat and calories. Like cocoa powder, it will also have a bitter taste and is generally used as an additive to other baked sweets, such as brownies, biscotti, and cookies. Once again, you should choose the unsweetened or sugar-free baking chocolates.

Dark chocolate is made from chocolate liquor and comes in two forms: bittersweet and semisweet. When selecting dark chocolates, there are several things that you need to consider. First, as already stated, make sure it is at least 70% cocoa. The darker the chocolate, the more antioxidants or polyphenols, specifically flavonoids, it will contain. Second, make sure it is made with cocoa butter, not from (hydrogenated) oils. One reason that chocolate may have a beneficial effect on cholesterol is that cocoa butter contains stearic acid and oleic acid. Oleic acid is a monounsaturated fat, which is a "good" fat that has been shown to decrease "bad" LDL cholesterol, while leaving the "good" HDL cholesterol alone. I use sugar-free or organic dark chocolates as a dip for a variety of nuts and fruits.

Other types of chocolates are semisweet chocolate, which is dark chocolate with added sugar and cocoa butter. Because of the additives, semisweet chocolate will contain less flavonols and more calories, than bittersweet dark chocolate. Milk chocolate is made from chocolate liquor, milk, sugar, and other ingredients. Because it is highly processed with other additives, it will have fewer healthy flavonols and will be higher in calories and saturated fats. Chocolate candy bars are usually made from milk chocolate and have so many additives, such as caramel, sugar, (partially) hydrogenated oils, etc., that they actually contain very little of healthier dark chocolate. If you must eat a candy bar, try to choose ones that are made of sugar-free dark chocolate, contain healthier additives, such as unsweetened coconut and nuts, and do not have (partially) hydrogenated oils. White chocolate does not contain chocolate liquor and many organizations, including the FDA, do not consider it to be a real chocolate. However, a quality white chocolate should contain cocoa butter, sugar, milk solids, vanilla, and lecithin. Although, it is made with cocoa butter, it will contain very little of the healthy flavonols. Some white chocolates are made with vegetable fat instead of cocoa butter and therefore, will be inferior in both taste and quality.

Researchers found that eating trans fats increased LDL "bad" cholesterol levels. Trans fats, the unhealthy fats, disappear from your body at the rate of 15% a year once you stop eating them (*Prevention*, April 2004, p. 72 and September 2004, p. 71).

Most fats and oils in our diets are composed of fat molecules known as long-chain triglycerides (LCTs). Coconut oil, however, is made up of predominately of medium chain triglycerides (MCTs). In one study, a group of normal-weight men ate a meal for breakfast that contained MCTs. Food intakes were then measured at lunch and dinner. Although the subjects ate less at lunch, they did not eat more at dinner, so total daily food intake decreased. This study found that when MCTs are eaten at one meal, hunger is forestalled and less food is eaten at the next (*Let's Live*, January 2005, pp. 64-65).

Chocolate is delicious and heart-healthy. A recent trial involving 45 subjects who consumed 75 grams daily of either white chocolate, dark chocolate, or dark chocolate enriched with cocoa polyphenols found the concentration of HDL "good" cholesterol increased in the dark chocolate groups by 11% and 14%, respectively. No effect was observed in the white chocolate group. A second finding showed a 12% decrease in LDL "bad" cholesterol levels in all three groups (*Let's Live*, February 2005, p. 20).

A new study found that rice bran oil has cholesterol-lowering properties. Researchers found that concentrations of certain compounds in the oil reduce lipid, fat, or fatty substances in the blood. To get the most heart healthy benefits, check the label to ensure it contains phytosterols, plant-based compounds known to reduce cholesterol. Rice bran oil has a high smoke point (490°), so it is great for frying as well as baking, salad dressings, and marinades (*Delicious Living*, July 2005, p. 20).

Spices/Seasonings & Beverages

Spices/Seasonings

Although, the UDSA 2005 My Pyramid does not have a specific category for spices/seasonings and beverages, the USDA does mention the importance of monitoring and limiting the daily intakes for two specific groups — salt/sodium and alcoholic beverages. In relation to spices/seasonings, the USDA stresses that your daily intake of salt and sodium should not exceed 2,400 mg and most nutritional labels use this number as the maximum limit of sodium intake per day, as well. However, it is important to note that one teaspoon of salt is approximately 2,000 mg of sodium. Remember my number one rule of shopping — read the labels, and try to purchase low-salt or no-salt products, whenever possible.

Some of the foods that contain the highest amounts of sodium are processed luncheon meats, cured meats, and soy sauce. Because many processed foods, from canned vegetables to spaghetti sauce, may contain a certain amount of sodium, it is almost never necessary to add salt while preparing meals. In almost all cases, people add salt out of habit. I used to add salt while preparing meals even though I had already added garlic salt or onion salt. Once I realized how much salt I was adding, I found it very easy to stop. With the exception of a few of my personal recipes, salt is not even an ingredient. I will on occasion use other types of seasoning mixes, such as *Tony Chachere's* original Creole seasoning, *Old Bay* seasoning, *Goya* seasonings, lemon pepper mix, which already contain salt. However, many regular seasonings, such as garlic powder, onion powder, and turmeric, will not contain salt, so this is where you must use your discretion when cooking.

At a meeting of the American Association Physiological Society, a preliminary study showed health benefits and medicinal properties of several spices. The antioxidants that spices contain may be beneficial in preventing free radical damage, which in turn may help to slow down and may prevent to onset of some diseases. For example, the East Indian spice curcumin, which gives curry spice tumeric its yellow color, may help protect the brain against Alzheimer's disease. Studies showed that curcumin triggers the production of the protein HO-1, which protected free radical damage in lab rats. Researchers believe that large-scale human studies will be necessary in order to determine the exact benefits of curcumin. Curcumin can also be found in turnips, brussel sprouts, and cauliflower.

Other spices which have shown health benefits include cardamom, which is an aromatic herb which tastes like black licorice, has been shown to ease the symptoms of indigestion. Cardamon is believed to help detoxify the body and to cleanse the liver. Cumin; which is used to spice up chili con carne and hot tamales, aids in the process of digestion and can ward off prostate cancer. Allicin; which is found in crushed garlic, when consumed in large quantities can help to reduce cholesterol and blood pressure, prevent weight gain, and some studies have shown that allicin may help prevent certain cancers. Fenugreek, which is a small seed used mostly in curry powders and for making pickles, has been shown to lower blood sugar levels in those with diabetes. Pepper is a known anti-oxidant with anti-bacterial effect which helps with digestion and weight loss because this spice stimulates the breakdown of fat cells.

Capsaicin, which is the main chemical in chili pepper, is known for its potent anti-inflammatory properties. It is also known to increase thermogenesis (heat production) and oxygen consumption which contributes to weight loss. This is a versatile spice, which can be used internally, as a spice, or externally as a topical cream to provide relief from the pain of arthritis. Just be very careful to wash your hands thoroughly after applying to your skin, as rubbing your eyes after applying the topical cream with capsaicin may create a burning sensation. Capsaicin has helped my husband whenever he feels the beginning of an asthma attack. Once he starts to experience the shortness of breath and his chest and throat tightening up, he will eat some green chili or red chili salsa. Within a few minutes, after sweating, his throat "loosens" up, his breathing becomes more regulated, and finally his throat "opens" up. So, I do not discount the health benefits that some spices may have.

In 2006, researchers from The University of Michigan Health System (UMHS), Department of Family Medicine found that the use of more herbs and spices and fewer traditional seasonings, such as sugar, salt, and fat, can help the overall health benefits and flavor of foods. They found that substituting herbs and spices in place of traditional seasonings helped to maintain a healthy weight, helped to prevent certain cancers, and even lowered blood pressure, control blood sugars and improved cardiovascular health. The UMHS researchers offered specific tips for picking and using herbs and spices to improve your overall health; which included reducing your daily intake of salt by using various herbs, such as oregano, thyme, rosemary, parsley, and garlic; use fresh garlic, as this helps to lower blood pressure and cholesterol; fight aging, help increase your memory by using rosemary; use basil, oregano, and rosemary to fight colds, as these herbs contain essential oils and antioxidants; drinking thyme as a tea aids those with chronic coughs; curcumin which gives curry its yellow color, contains tumeric, has anti-inflammatory properties which has been shown to shrink pre-cancerous lesions or colon polyps and acts in a similar way as non-steroidal anti-inflammatory drugs; the use of "warming spices," like ginger, nutmeg, cinnamon, allspice, pepper, cayenne peppers and others helps to decrease blood pressure by dispersing blood throughout the body more evenly; and finally, the use of ginger helps with a stomach ache by decreasing the oxidative products in your digestive tract than cause nausea.

What I found was that some of their tips were things both my husband and I were already doing. For example, we already substituted many of the herbs and spices for salt; we use garlic in almost every dish we prepare; we use rosemary when we cook any type of fish; whenever we make stir-fry dishes we almost always use a curry sauce; and we used the various "warming spices" in a lot of our meals from breakfast, in oatmeal, to desserts, in our pie crusts and pie fillings. I am sure that many of you already use some of these various herbs and spices. It is just a matter of trying to be more inclusive in expanding the use of more herbs and spices in many more of the dishes you prepare for yourself and your family.

Beverages

Without any doubt, water is still the best beverage option to choose and is calorie-free. Not only does water keep your body from dehydrating, it plays a major role in almost every body function, from cushioning the joints to bringing oxygen to body cells and removing waste from the body. It is recommended that the average adult drink eight 8 oz. glasses of water a day or a total of 64 ounces of water a day. Although, this may sound like an extremely large amount of water, once you actually measure 8 ounces in a glass, you will find that it is not as much a you think it is and it will therefore be easier to get this recommended amount into your daily routine. Lastly, do not be rigid about the thought of drinking water. You can work yourself up to the required amount by adding a one glass of water at lunch and dinner, then increasing the amount at each meal. I usually drink two - 16 ounce glasses of water with my lunch and dinner. Also, I drink at least an 8 ounce glass of water upon returning from my daily walks and hikes, thus meeting the recommended 64 ounces of water a day.

However, if you feel you cannot drinks 64 ounces of water a

day, there are other beverage options available for you to choose. Many soft drinks are now available that are both sugar free and caffeine free. Also, there are many sugar free powdered drink mixes available, that are specifically targeted for those people that are on special diets, such as diabetics. However, you must still be careful to not overindulge and drink too much of these products. Ingesting large amounts of sugar substitutes can lead to other minor health problems, such as diarrhea and upset stomach. Do not lock yourself up in a small box. Many times we get caught up in "comfort products," which simply means that eating or drinking these products make us feel better, they bring us comfort. Try to find new comfort products that are more natural healthier choices. As for my own personal preference, a nice cold glass of water is my "comfort" beverage.

There is growing evidence of health benefits associated with the antioxidants found in coffee and regular teas. Coffee provides more antioxidants than any other beverage. The antioxidants in coffee are polyphenols, which may prevent some cancers and reduce the risks of developing Type 2 Diabetes and heart disease. However, coffee acts as a diuretic, which has a dehydrating effect on your body, Because of this it should be consumed in moderation, limiting your coffee consumption to no more than 2-4 cups per day, and coffee should never count toward your daily eight - 8 ounce glasses of water recommendation. Also, coffee does contain caffeine, which can make people nervous and jittery. Lastly, coffee does not contain the other healthy nutrients, such as vitamins, minerals, and fiber, which are found in grains, fruits, and vegetables.

Because of the fermentation process, Oolong and black teas are higher in the antioxidants, theaflavins and thearubigins. While white and green teas, which are less processed, are higher in the antioxidant catechin. Similar to coffee, studies on tea indicate that drinking tea may prevent some types of cancers, lower cholesterol levels, and delay the onset of Type 2 Diabetes. Although, studies are still ongoing as to the exact benefits of drinking tea, most researchers agree that it is safe to drink at least 2 cups a day. On the other hand, herbal teas, which are not really a tea but infusions of various herbs, flowers, and spices, may help to strengthen the immune system. Different herbs and herbal combinations help the body recover from multiple illnesses and conditions, such as PMS, menopause, headaches, and cold and flu symptoms.

Farhad Islami, a research fellow, along with other researchers at Tehran University of Medical Sciences conducted several "tea" studies in the northern province of Golestan in Iran. Golestan, was unique, in that this area had a much higher percentage of esophageal cancer, despite the fact that they do not drink alcoholic beverages or smoke. Both of these habits are found to be direct links to this particular type of cancer in other parts of the world. In the first case-controlled study, they compared 300 people with esophageal cancer to 571 people who were cancer-free. The study found that those with this cancer were more likely to drink tea, at very high temperatures, more regularly than those who did not have cancer. One part of this study asked the participants two questions: 1) if they drank their tea lukewarm, warm, hot, or very hot and 2) how long they waited after pouring their tea before drinking it. In the second study, the researchers asked the general population of Golestan, approximately 50,000 participants, these same two questions and then measured the actual temperature of the tea as it cooled. This provided the researchers with information as to how accurate the participants were in determining the temperature of their tea and also provided information which linked the temperature of the tea to those with esophageal cancer.

The major link between tea and developing esophageal cancer was not linked to drinking tea, but to the temperature of the tea. The hotter the temperature of the tea, over 60 degrees centigrade, the more likely those in the Golestan Province developed this type of cancer. The researchers deduced several theories on why this appears to happen. First, very hot drinks (not only tea, but all hot beverages) might irritate the esophagus, causing inflammation, which in turn begin the process that damage the cells and increase the risk of cancer. Second, any hot liquid can also damage the lining of the esophagus, thereby allowing cancer-causing substances from other sources to find their way into these damaged cells. These cancer-causing substances can come from various sources in our diets, including but not limited to substances from charred foods that have been grilled, or more likely, from cigarette smoke. In Golestan, those who drank their tea hot to very hot also smoked opium, which is a common habit in the region. The major recommendation from this study is if you drink coffee, tea, or any type of hot beverage, take the time to let your beverage cool before enjoying the drink! This way you get the health benefits from the drink and avoid damaging the esophagus.

Shortly after my father passed away, my younger sister called me because she wanted to try an herbal capsule, called jiaogulan. She had read that this was supposed to help rejuvenate her skin, help reduce wrinkles, and help regulate her sleeping pattern. She wanted to know if I had ever heard of it and if I would recommend her taking it. Since I never heard of it, I told her to wait until I researched this herbal supplement. Then I went on a massive internet search looking for any and all information, and specifically research-related information, about this herb. What I found compelled me to try it for myself. Jiaogulan (pronounced jow — goo — lawn) is known in China as the "Immortality Herb" and is believed to contain numerous rejuvenating properties. According to various studies, the use of jiaogulan has shown promise in several areas, which include the regulation of serum cholesterol, triglycerides, LDL and HDL levels, in helping to maintain healthy blood pressure levels, in improving and strengthening digestion, in increasing strength and endurance, and in supporting the immune system. Also, the studies found that this herb has both adaptogenic and antioxidant properties. The adaptogenic properties have a biphasic effect on brain functions, which allows your body to adapt and cope with stress, thereby building a natural resistance to stress. While the antioxidant properties in jiaogulan protect against free radical damage.

Jiaogulan contains four types of saponins exactly like those found in Panax ginseng and seventeen types of saponins similar to those found in the same ginseng. Ultimately scientists found as many as eighty-two types of saponins in jiaogulan, while ginseng has as many as twenty-eight. So jiaogulan has three to four times the saponins than ginseng. These saponins, known as gypenosides in jiaogulan, are the reason many believe that this herb has the ability to have the regulatory effect on a number of the body's systems. Jiaogulan can be easily found in supplement form, although I read that the herb is very hard to standardize and the effects can vary. So I looked for it in other forms and found it at a local vitamin/grocery store in an herbal tea, which carry this tea under the scientific name of gynostemma pentaphyllum or simply gynostemma.

As it stated on the box, you should have one to two cups of the tea at night. I found that my body adapted to this tea quickly and that I could actually feel this tea working. No sooner than I went to bed, I fell asleep within a few minutes, slept through the night, and woke up almost eight hours to the minute. Within a few days of starting this tea, I found a way to virtually eliminate the occurrence of my nightly hot flashes and get a good night's sleep. Because I am now sleeping well, I wake up more relaxed and less anxious. This particular tea has helped to alleviate the nightly aches and pain I feel that are associated with my diagnosis of fibromyalgia. Also, I feel energized enough to want to exercise. I feel that this particular tea has helped relieve my restlessness, pain, anxiety, and mild depression more than anything else I have tried.

The controversy of alcoholic beverage consumption is growing because some recent studies suggest that some compounds in these beverages, specifically wine and beer, may actually have some health benefits. According to the American Cancer Society, while several recent studies have found that moderate consumption of red wine (two to three glasses a day) may decrease your risk for developing heart disease and lung cancer, moderate amounts of red wine may also increase your the risk for developing certain cancers, such as breast, colorectal, and intestinal. While numerous studies are still ongoing and as more information becomes available, there is still the fact that many alcoholic beverages are very high in calories. As mentioned earlier, the key to eating fruits and vegetables is that they should be nutrient-dense, meaning the nutritional values found in the food outweigh the calories of the food. This is the same approach you should use when consuming any alcoholic beverage and these types of beverages are simply not nutrient-dense, they are calorie-dense. So once again, the USDA stresses that the key to adding any type of alcoholic beverage to your meal is moderation and strict limits.

A USDA study found that people cut their mildly elevated cholesterol levels by 7% and their LDL "bad" cholesterol by 11% after three weeks of drinking 5-daily cups of black tea. It is recommended that you drink at least two-four cups of tea daily (*Prevention*, March 2004, p. 44).

Red wine contains resveratrol, a compound found in the skins of red grapes, which blocks a key protein that cancer cells need to survive. Red wine also contains cholesterol fighters, saponins, which protects the heart by trapping cholesterol before it can be absorbed into the bloodstream. These two compounds in red vintages may provide an answer to lower heart disease risks. Saponin levels are three to 10 times higher in red wines than in white wines. One glass of red wine 3−4 times a week is recommended. Resveratrol is also found in raspberries and peanuts (*Prevention*, March, 2004, p. 44 and November 2004, p. 80).

A USDA study showed that cinnamon may be able to lower your cholesterol, triglycerides, and blood sugar levels by 12%-30% in 40 days. Cinnamon makes the muscle and liver cells more sensitive to signals from insulin. It is recommended that you have ½ teaspoon daily (*Prevention*, June 2004, p. 50).

Dark beer is richer in the healthy plant chemicals, polyphenols, than lighter beers. Polyphenols stop platelets, which are the building blocks of clots, from sticking together in the blood (*Prevention*, October 2004, p. 84).

Recent findings show that the polyphenols in green tea can protect against cancer and may even destroy cancer cells. A new study suggests that another component in green tea, epigallocatechin-3-gallate, may kill cells of the most common form of leukemia.

Although it's too soon to recommend drinking green tea to prevent or treat leukemia, researchers say that drinking more of it isn't harmful and may offer other benefits due to its antioxidant content (*Let's Live*, December 2004, 12).

The active compound silymarin, found in milk thistle, lessens the damaging effects of alcohol on your liver. Although this herb is safe for regular use, some people initially experience mild stomach upset. The recommended daily dose is 150 to 200 mg two to three times daily. Capsules should be standardized to 70%-80% silymarin (*Prevention*, December 2004, p. 39).

The yellow pigment in turmeric, curcumin, reduces the action of a number of genes that promote inflammation, which is linked to heart disease, colon cancer, and Alzheimer's. Turmeric, found mostly in East Indian recipes, is found in curry spice (*Newsweek*, January 17, 2005, 48).

Greens with a vinaigrette before a starchy meal may help control your blood sugar. Vinegar contains acetic acid, which may inactivate certain starch-digesting enzymes, slowing carbohydrate digestion (*Prevention*, February 2005, p. 44).

Obesity in the United States continues to increase. According to a study Americans now consume 200 to 300 more calories a day than they consumed 30 years ago. Approximately, one-third to one-half of those calories is in high-fructose corn syrup, the sweetener in all sugar-based soft drinks (*Natural Health*: Special Issue, Summer 2005, p. 9).

Miscellaneous Information

Although much of the additional information from magazine articles that was listed above was placed within the appropriate food group or category, some can and often does apply to multiple categories. As in the cases of the following information, I found these to be useful in helping to guide my food choices. Many times I found that by reading some of the articles, especially from multiple sources, this further builds on the fact that many different studies from reputable sources provided the foundation needed in order to live a healthier lifestyle. In the end, with this information I will continue to build a stronger knowledge base for the healthier way of eating that I now enjoy.

Some ingredients in traditional Italian pizza, including tomato (which contain lycopene) and olive oil, may protect the heart. Italian pizzas are usually made of thin wheat flour crusts, fresh herbs and a small amount of mozzarella. The study found that those who ate one 7-oz serving of Italian-style pizza per week reduced the risk of having a heart attack by 38% and two 7-oz servings per week reduced the risk by 56% (*Let's Live*, November 2004, p. 14).

Selenium is a trace element found in meats, grains, seafood and some nuts, of which Brazil nuts contain the highest amount. Researchers analyzed data from three randomized trials and found a correlation between those with the highest levels of selenium in the blood had a 34% decreased risk of colorectal cancer compared with those with the lowest levels of selenium. While researchers only assessed blood levels of selenium derived from food, supplements are available. The daily recommended dietary allowance (RDA) is 70 mcg for men and 55 mcg for women (*Let's Live*, February 2005, p. 21).

Lipoic acid is found a number of food sources, including dark green leafy vegetables (such as spinach and collard greens), broccoli, meat, brewer's yeast, and wheat germ. A number of studies found using lipoic acid may prevent and lower high blood pressure and insulin resistance. In one study, the blood sugar concentration in patients was reduced by almost 10 percent after 12 weeks of treatment with lipoic acid. In another, it prevented increases in glucose, triglycerides, free fatty acids, insulin, and insulin resistance (in fructose-fed rats) and improved insulin sensitivity (*Health Smart Today*, Summer 2005, pp. 36-37).

Folate, which is found in whole grains, leafy greens, and orange juice, may protect you against bowel cancer. In a study of people with pre-cancerous polyps (precursors to bowel cancer), supplementing with folic acid (400 mcg daily) actually reversed a process that healthy cells use to deactivate certain genes, but is usually out of control in tumor cells. Too little folate may induce this process and thereby increase the possibility of growths becoming cancerous. As a supplement take 400 mcg of folic acid daily (*Let's Live*, August 2005, p. 18).

Miscellaneous Herbal and Home Remedies

Many health food stores carry information related to herbal preparations and their uses. Another good source of information about herbal teas and their uses may be elderly family members. Many of our elders grew up using herbal preparations to treat a multitude of conditions. Within some families, there are remedies that are passed down from one generation to the next. For example, I remember my mother making a cup of *canela* (cinnamon stick tea) for me to drink whenever I had an upset stomach. Today, there are many types of specialty herbal teas on the market that are formulated toward specific problems, such as PMS, menopause-relief, asthma-relief, anxiety, and flu and cold symptoms.

My husband has his own personal remedies that he learned from his mother, as well. For example he discovered his own remedy for treating and alleviating the pain and redness associated with less severe cases of sunburn. First, he applies a liberal amount of aloe vera lotion to the sunburned area, making sure to get complete coverage. Because the skin is both dry and damaged, it will naturally soak up the lotion. He then applies coconut oil. This is repeated as many times as needed, for several days. In most cases, this helps prevent further damage to the skin and even peeling, if the sunburn is not severe.

Another one of his home remedies is treating an insect sting. Recently, while weeding, I was stung by a scorpion, a non-poisonous type that is native to the southwest area. While these scorpion stings are not fatal, the sting itself is very painful and the area can swell. My husband simply mixed baking soda with water to make a soft, watery paste and placed my finger in the paste. The baking soda will draw the "poison" out of the wound and decrease the pain and any possible swelling. Within a half hour the pain subsided, although I had slight swelling within the area for the rest of the day. Basically, home remedies and even herbal remedies can and do come in handy at certain times. So, at times it may pay to take the advice that your elders and older family members may give you.

In a 2001 study, researchers from Georgetown University found that Oil of Oregano protected against certain fungi. The particular oil of oregano to use is the one that comes from the Origanum Vulgare plant, also known as Mediterranean Wild Oregano. This particular wild, mountain-grown variety has low levels (less than 2%) of thymol, which is an anti-microbial compound with known toxicity at higher levels. However, thymol is also a known immune booster. Mediterranean wild oregano also contains a number of phenols, of which carvarcol being the most potent. Carvarcol is a known anti-viral, anti-fungal, anti-bacterial, and anti-parasitic compound. These two antioxidants, thymol and carvarcol, act as free radical scavengers, which help protect the body from free radical damage. Oil of Oregano can be used internally or externally, which makes this oil a very versatile herbal treatment. Although a skeptic at first, the lead researcher found during his study that this particular herbal remedy helped treat his sinus infection, when other more conventional drugs failed to work.

During this past winter, I felt the beginning of a severe cold and flu that my husband passed to onto me. While he was ill, he prepared an herb drink to help ease the effects of the virus. This drink helped to lessen the effects of the virus and the length of the virus, as well. He researched some herbal remedies for colds and flu and found some very interesting suggestions. He found that wild oil of oregano has both anti-bacterial and anti-viral properties. He simply placed 4 drops of the oil of oregano in 1—4 ounces of warm water and drank this mixture. While the oil of oregano is bitter and provides a mild warm and burning sensation, like wasabi, this sensation goes away after approximately 1 minute. To help ease this sensation, after a few minutes, if I still felt the bitterness, I then drank some juice or regular water. However, drinking this mixture three times a day, helped to ease the major symptoms I suffered from and reduced the overall length of my cold.

The astringent tannins in distilled witch hazel significantly ease sunburn symptoms by reducing inflammation, redness and pain (*Prevention*, July 2004, p. 34).

Smelling lavender oil may blur the memory of pain. Researchers exposed more than 13 men and 13 women to uncomfortable heat and pressure on muscles in the jaw and back and then had them inhale lavender or an odorless control for 10 minutes during different sessions. The lavender oil significantly reduced the memory of pain's intensity and unpleasantness. Shake 5 to 10 drops of lavender essential oil onto a tissue and inhale freely during a potentially painful procedure, such as dental work (*Prevention*, January 2005, p. 46).

Limonene, an ingredient in citrus and some other plants, may "burn" away inhaled ozone that can increase inflammation in the lungs and produce symptoms of asthma. In a promising recent study, rats with asthma showed no signs of the disease after inhaling citrus aromas (*Let's Live*, March 2005, p. 25).

The aloe vera leaf eases the pain and speeds healing by increasing blood supply and oxygen to and injury, which helps the body repair damaged tissues. The aloe vera leaf contains a gel with 75 potentially active substances, including antioxidants, amino acids, and enzymes, is a proven antibacterial and anti-inflammatory (*Prevention*, August 2005, p. 98).

The Importance of Exercise

As in most diet plans, in order to be successful, you must increase your level of physical activity and engage in some form of exercise. This is just as important as eating properly within the major food groups. And as with the food groups, this generally requires that you add or even increase the amount of physical activity you engage in. Before you change or add to any exercise plan, you should always seek the advice of your personal physician. This is what my psychology professor insisted on before I undertook my personal experiment in my college behavior modification course and this is what I advise you to do as well. Your doctor can guide you as to what types of exercise you can safely begin with and monitor your health throughout your exercise regimen.

Recommended USDA daily physical activity requirements:

❖   Moderate or vigorous physical activity for at least 30 minutes a day.

Moderate exercise does not include your regular daily activities, such as walking around the house, to and from your car, etc. To properly engage in moderate exercise you must walk briskly at the rate of 3-4 miles within an hour, dance (not slow dance), or take up general lightweight training, become involved in hiking, or even gardening and yard work. The key to moderate exercise is to try to get your heart rate going. There are many ways to incorporate moderate exercise into your lifestyle. You could, for example, join a power-walking club at a mall. These clubs usually meet before the mall opens. Many malls that sponsor walking clubs have mile markings along the inside perimeter of the mall. This way, as you exercise you can also keep track how far you have actually walked. You could also take what you normally do and just step it up a bit, as in the case of golfing. When you golf, do not use a cart and, more importantly, walk and carry your own clubs. For myself, I do not always take the closest parking space when I go to a large store or mall. I will sometimes park a little farther away and briskly walk to the mall or store entrance. If the weather and time of day permits, and always keeping your safety in mind, you could walk in one entrance and then leave from another and briskly walk the outer perimeter of the mall back to your car.

Vigorous exercise, steps it up yet another notch, and would include activities such as, running or jogging about 5-6 miles an hour, power-walking at 4-5 miles an hour, aerobics, swimming, or bicycling. Also, any exercise, such as basketball, football, moderate to heavy weightlifting, advanced yoga, and even heavy yard work would count as vigorous. This type of exercise generally includes resistance, strength building, and weight-bearing activities, along with a more intense aerobic workout. Vigorous exercise can build on whichever type of moderate exercise you choose and can be very instrumental in weight loss.

The key is to find whatever exercise program or the type of physical activity that works for you, within your own limits. By this I mean that you need to consider the amount of time and any and all health-related conditions you may have. This is important because both of these factors will determine what types of exercise programs you will be able to incorporate into your lifestyle.

For example, although I know I would like to incorporate higher intensity workouts more than I currently do, I have to take into consideration that, in addition to having elevated blood triglyceride levels, I also have "bad" knees. In the fall of 1998, while moving furniture and painting my living room, I attempted to "dead lift" a five-gallon container of paint. After hearing my left knee pop and experiencing ongoing residual pain for several weeks in both my knees, my doctor referred me to a physical therapist, with a diagnosis of chondromalacia patella. This is simply a condition in which the cartilage in my kneecaps is slowing softening, which at some point may require surgery. Although my left knee was worse, my right knee was not much better. After reviewing my options, the therapist worked with me to fashion several exercise programs that would help to rehabilitate and improve my overall knee strength and delay the need for immediate knee surgery. He also guided me to the type of schedule I would need to follow. Because he suggested low impact exercises he wanted me to briskly walk on a treadmill. I later substituted the Gazelle, because it is a no to low impact training machine, for about 15—20 minutes, three times a week. Currently, the only thing I need to ensure is that I make the time to follow a regular exercise program at least three times a week or take my dog for a 3—5 mile walk or hike every day.

Another example is the type of physical activity my husband tried to incorporate into his schedule. For the past twenty-five years, he has been living with moderate to severe lower back pain because of a car accident. Because his right leg was shattered in the accident, he was advised that he could only engage in low impact exercises, such as brisk walking and hiking. Also, his back pain increases if he stands or sits for long periods of time. After years of trying different types of exercises that were supposed to alleviate the pain and strengthen his back muscles, he found that they could not ease the pain for any extended period of time. Then he saw a *Tony Little Gazelle* exercise machine at a department store and jokingly remarked about the inventor. After trying the machine for five minutes, his back muscles started to relax and that night his pain was not as bothersome. The next day he went back to the store and tried the machine again, and found that his back felt even better. His third trip to the store is when he decided to purchase this exercise machine. Although this may sound like a "Tony Little infomercial testimonial," in his case 15—30 minutes on the Gazelle at least three times a week has virtually eliminated his lower back pain. This has encouraged him to add moderate weightlifting into his schedule, as well. So he not only found a workable exercise program that easily fits into his lifestyle, he found one that he enjoys. Because we both enjoy the exercise programs we engage in, exercising is not a chore.

According to a new study, women who exercise and are more physically fit than average have blood that is less likely to clot and therefore have a lower risk of heart attacks. An enzyme made by the body that breaks up blood clots was higher in physically fit women than in unfit women. In addition, a marker that indicates blood clot creation was lower in fit women, suggesting that people who exercise may be better able to prevent the formation of blood clots which may be why exercisers are less likely to have heart attacks than people who do not exercise (*Health Smart Today*, Summer 2005, p. 22).

A new study of 139 women ages 20 to 35 found that those who

took a 45-minute step aerobics class three times a week for 6 months increased bone mineral density in their spines, legs, and heels up to 3%. Step aerobics may be even better than ace bone enhancers, such as jumping rope and jogging, because it includes more changes in direction and speed, which, along with impact, stimulate bone growth (*Prevention*, August 2005, p. 37).

Researchers found that a 40—50 minute *Pilates* workout can burn calories as well as aerobic workouts. Based on a 150 lb. woman, on average, a 40—50 minute basic workout burned 200 calories; an intermediate 292 calories; and an advanced 360 calories (*Prevention*, August 2005, p. 46).

Miscellaneous Health

An important part of my journey to health and wellness was the fact that I continually learn new facts about health and wellness, in general. As with my journey in my healthy eating plan and my exercise plan, I have to follow a journey in my medical plan, as well. Because the area of medicine and health is ever changing and developing there will always be newer, updated advice and advances in this important area. For example, in 2007 the limits for the optimal total, LDL, and HDL cholesterol levels were changed and updated. Because the new acceptable levels were lowered within all cholesterol levels, this placed more people on cholesterol-lowering drugs than before. Another medical change that occurred was within the thyroid-stimulating hormone (TSH) test, which determines whether you may have hypothyroidism, which is simply a struggling and under active thyroid. The new test result parameters now include many more people that were previously determined to have normal thyroid test result. This also has the impact to place even more people on thyroid medication. So, it is important that you as an individual know about changes that may have a direct effect on your overall health maintenance plan and about tests and results of tests that can determine whether or not you will join the ranks of people placed on prescription medication.

Researchers found that total cholesterol (TC) will naturally go up in winter and down in summer. In a study of 517 people, their cholesterol was checked several times in a year. The seasonal variation put 22% of the patients over the official high-cholesterol mark of 240mg/dl when tested in winter. Blood contains less water in winter, slightly concentrating cholesterol. It is recommended that you get several checks during the year, with at least one in the spring or fall, when levels are at a midpoint (*Prevention*, October 2004, p. 54).

A recent study found a clear link between hostility, anger, and depression and increased levels of C-reactive protein (CRP), a marker of inflammation in the blood. CRP, a protein that is released in the body in response to stress and other threats to the immune system, contributes to heart disease. Healthy adults who had mild to moderate symptoms of depression, anger, or hostility were found to have CRP levels that were two to three times higher than those of their calmer counterparts. Also, the more negative the mood, the higher the CRP levels. Once elevated, CRP levels tend to stay consistently high, which may lead to increased narrowing of the arteries and subsequent heart disease (*Health Smart Today*, Spring 2005, p. 14).

A 15-year study has shown a correlation between eating fast food, gaining weight, and insulin resistance. A recent study found that as fast-food consumption increases, the risk of obesity and Type 2 Diabetes increases. Those who consumed fast food two or more times per week gained about 10 more pounds during the study and had twice the increase in insulin resistance as those who consumed fast food less than once per week (*Diabetic Living*, Summer 2005, p. 20).

If you have trouble sleeping you may have a predisposition to diabetes. A 15-year study of more than 6,000 men found that those who had a difficult time falling or staying asleep were more likely to develop diabetes. This study indicates that problems with sleeping may contribute to glucose intolerance, impaired insulin function, and increased risk for diabetes (*Diabetic Living*, Summer 2005, p. 20).

Researchers found that regular sleep loss is associated with higher body mass index. The study showed that those who slept only five hours, well below the recommended eight hours, had elevated amounts of ghrelin, a hormone that triggers appetite, and reduced leptin, a hormone that tells your body when it's full. So the less you sleep, the more you may weigh (*Delicious Living*, July 2005, p. 20).

Researchers in Canada have found that people who live in neighborhoods with a lot of fast-food outlets are more likely to get heart disease. In the Toronto-based study, investigators analyzed the number of fast-food outlets per capita in 380 areas of the province of Ontario and found that a higher density of fast-food restaurants increases risk for heart disease, regardless of other health factors or income levels (*Let's Live*, October 2005, p. 20).

Researchers measured blood vessel inflammation levels, using the C-reactive protein (CRP) test. Those who got less than 50% of the RDA (310 to 420 mg per day) for the magnesium were almost 3 times as likely to have dangerously high CRP levels as those who consumed enough. Being over age 40 and overweight and consuming less than 50% of the RDA more than doubled the risk of blood-vessel damaging inflammation. Some food rich in magnesium are soy, beans, seeds, whole grains, bananas, dried apricots, avocadoes, and dark green leafy vegetables (*Prevention*, November 2005, p. 78).

5

Diet and Tradition

I f you do not understand what is traditional for you and your family, you cannot understand why it is important to want to keep certain foods part of your healthy diet. For some it may take a little research into your preferences, but for others it will be effortless. Because I did not really have a lot of hard knowledge about my culture, I needed to do a lot more research and reading about what I wanted to include. First, I used a lot of traditional family recipes handed down to me from family members and worked to improve them. This allowed me to build a foundation of staple meals that I wanted to include in my diet. Then as I began to research other "traditional" foods of my culture, I was able to make my foundation of staple foods more extensive. So, as I researched some of the things I wanted to know about the basic foods I had thought of including in my personal diet, I realized that many of the foods were already part of my tradition and culture. This is something that you may find true for yourself, as well.

From the beginning of our journey, my husband was more interested in trying to incorporate many "native" foods back into our diet than I was. While I found that incorporating more "native" foods would be interesting, I was very comfortable with both the base knowledge of family recipes that I had accumulated over the years and with my husband's recipes he shared with me. Also, I was a little apprehensive about adding "native" foods in my diet. After all, I was raised in Chicago, and although I have been in the southwest since 1993, I did not want the idea of adding more "native" foods to be at the expense of removing other foods I enjoyed. On the other hand, my husband was fascinated by the fact that many of our combined traditional foods contained many health benefits. Ultimately, for the both of us, the foods that represent our combined cultures and traditions are important. This is why he wanted to include some of our traditional foods in this section. For him, it is important that you and your family realize the impact of your culture and traditions in your diet and in the way you cook.

Understanding and Embracing the Foods of Our Cultures

Understanding the traditional foods of indigenous Mexican and Great Lakes cultures begins by going back in time, and I don't mean back to your grandmother's time, but way back. Since my husband is a cultural anthropologist, he researched the diet of Native North Americans prior to the arrival of Europeans. Although the foods Indigenous Americans ate varied widely, populations both agricultural and hunter-gatherer had diets that were high in fiber, and of course made up of whole unprocessed foods. For my people, from the Mexican state of Durango, a diet based on whole stone ground corn also included fruits, greens known as *quelites*, squash, beans, various kinds of chiles, *nopales* (prickly pear cactus pads), nuts, wild vegetables and tubers, wild game, and some freshwater fish. In fact, before the Europeans arrived Mexican food was very healthy indeed! But the Mexican food we see today is full of fatty meats, lard, cheese, and processed flour. It is a far cry from what my ancestors ate.

For my husband, his indigenous ancestors in the Great Lakes region consumed a wide variety of both cultivated and gathered foods, along with wild game, and lots of freshwater fish. Among some of the more prominent foods were wild rice, corn, beans, squash, wild vegetables and tubers, nuts, blueberries, blackberries, raspberries, strawberries, many other kinds of wild fruit, maple syrup, mushrooms, venison, moose, turkey, and a wide variety of fresh water fish. In addition, people of the Great Lakes had an almost endless variety of plants that were used for seasoning and teas. My husband tells me that there are stories of people in the Great Lakes being very long-lived before the arrival of the Europeans.

When I began to really look at the traditional Native diets of my people and his, certain themes emerged, foods such as beans, corn, squash, nuts, wild game, freshwater fish and fruits were common to both. My people differed in that chiles and nopales were used regularly, and his ancestors had eaten wild rice, maple syrup, and many berries not known to the Tepehuanes. Also, our combined dietary histories included high fiber whole foods that were low in saturated fats. When my husband had finished exploring the history of our foods and how they were gathered, I realized even more than ever that we had to increase the fiber in our diets, and we also needed to be more physically active. If either of us were going to beat the genetic cards we had been dealt, we had to make these changes. However, I was very happy about the fact that I really liked all the foods from our distant collective past. I was also happy that I would not have to give up my beans, tortillas and chiles because they, like real Mexican food, were and are healthy.

Beyond the obvious fact that eating mostly unprocessed or minimally processed foods with more fiber is good for me, I like the fact that I am doing something that does not ask me to turn away from my cultural past. At times I can even picture in my mind my great great-grandmother leaning over a *metate* (corn grinding stone) making the *masa* (dough) for tortillas, the same corn tortillas that have sustained my people for thousands of years. For my husband it is a little easier. He actually did go out in the woods as a youth and young adult to pick wild fruits and collect plants for medicinal use. He also fished, and at times hunted. Finally, his mother grew a variety of seasonal vegetables in her backyard garden. Still, for each of us, honoring the past and modifying what we do to fit our present lifestyle gives me a sense that we have built on our indigenous heritage instead of abandoning our roots to follow a cookie cutter diet plan designed by someone who doesn't take into account who we are as people, as cultural beings.

Besides, how can you ask Indigenous Americans to give up corn? Corn is more than food to us. It is sacred. Important rituals for many of the first peoples of Canada, Mexico, and the United States included prayers for corn, which in the U.S. Southwest even involved sacred corn meal. Corn is something that is not just in my diet, it is in my soul. The same is true for the importance of wild rice to his people. The indigenous people of the Western Great Lakes have a belief that they were guided to what is now Northern Michigan, Wisconsin, and Minnesota by the creator who had told them their long journey to find a home would end when they got to "the place where the food grows on the water." Wild rice comes from an indigenous grass of the Western Great Lakes region where it grows in shallow lakes. Imagine being asked to give up such an important part of your culinary heritage to follow a generic "one diet fits all" type of plan that cannot embrace different cultures and traditions. You would always feel left out at family gatherings and what you ate would have little connection to the person you are.

However, you do not have to be Native American to follow what I have written in this book. All of us have a cultural heritage and family tradition, whether it is from the Americas, Europe, Asia, Africa, Australia, or the Pacific Basin. What is important is that we all explore our distant past in terms of food. What did your ancestors eat before industrialization and the switch to highly processed readymade foods? People worldwide had diets that were higher in fiber. So, you may not have a cultural background that includes tortillas, but if you dig deep and do your research, you will likely find that many of your modern recipes that are based in your cultural tradition have evolved from an older and more wholesome form. This is especially true for breads. Breads in ancient times, almost without exception, were made from whole grains. This means that you could take your recipes for bread back to their whole grain roots. By doing this you will honor your past and take a step toward a healthier future at the same time.

Looking at Your Dietary Influences

For both my husband and me, we have used our cultural roots as a guide and built our way of eating on that foundation. Yes, tortillas, wild rice, beans, nuts, squash, turkey, chiles, and other native fruits and vegetables form the foundation of what we eat, but we have also incorporated rice, oats, wheat, broccoli, miso, chicken and dozens of other things that are not part of our collective cultural culinary past. Although, what we have done is to follow the basic concepts of eating a mostly plant-based diet with foods high in fiber, low in saturated fat, and as close to whole food as possible. Also, when we do alter foods or recipes, we tend to add foods or ingredients that are higher in fiber, replace saturated fats with good healthier fats, and replace red meats with chicken, turkey, or fish.

Developing a healthy diet is not just good for your health. It can be fun too. By exploring your past, you will be able to understand what your ancestors ate and why. Also, you will be able to preserve some of your history, and take pride in eating foods that you know some distant relative of yours had prepared way back when. Food, diet, and culture are tied together in a long braid that reaches back into the mist of time. What you do today may likely become the time-honored tradition of your descendents many years from now. So honor the old ways and the ancient ones, and add some of your own innovations in cooking to create a healthy way of living from today forward.

After reading several books on health, diet, and exercise, I found myself believing the reason many of these programs did not work for me was exactly what I thought. Many diet/weight loss programs do take into consideration your culture—whether you are Native-American, Mexican-American, Greek, Italian, Irish, etc.; your traditions—my family tradition of eating included many different traditional meals combined with foods that were non-traditional, which became part of our family tradition; and lastly your specific lifestyle preferences—whether or not you are a carnivore, omnivore, vegetarian, or vegan. Part of initiating the Seventh Step, in you developing your own healthy eating plan according to your culture, traditions, and personal lifestyle preferences, is understanding what you and your family wants to include in your particular situation.

If you want to use the USDA 2005 MyPyramid as a general guide, then use it to begin setting up you own healthy way of eating that fits you and your family. While, many health advocates still find some fault with the new and improved MyPyramid, others find this a useful tool to establish healthy eating habits. Some critics state that the pyramid gives too much duplicate information, such as the recommendation of 3 glasses of milk regardless of the age, gender, and exercise level differences for those who look to this pyramid for dietary advice. So while this may be a good starting point, you will ultimately need to make the choices that best suit you and your family. Many leading health organizations have adapted this pyramid and there are variations of the "pyramid" which provide a general guide for different ethnic and cultural groups. In doing internet searches, I found various food pyramids based on ethnicity, lifestyle, and medical conditions. For example, there are food pyramids which focus on Native Americans, Latin Americans, Asian Americans, and African Americans. Also, there are food pyramids for people who choose to be vegetarian and vegan, and even a Diabetic Food Pyramid.

Culture-Based Research in Diet and Disease

Because the growing number of those with "lifestyle" diseases, such as obesity and Type 2 Diabetes, many communities are now taking measures through education and prevention, and management of disease. Traditional methods to control "lifestyle" diseases failed in Mexican-American communities, in part to the substantial number of uninsured, non-English speaking individuals that need medical care. Because Mexican-Americans have one of the highest rates of obesity and Type 2 Diabetes, a time-limited grassroots community-based effort was developed in Dallas, Texas to address the needs of this community. This effort, which began in July 2003 and ended in March 2005, within the community included the collaboration with State of Texas, Department of Health and the Ruth Collins Diabetes Center (RCDC) at Baylor University Medical Center in Dallas. This collaboration developed a culturally appropriate intervention, known as the Community Diabetes Education (CoDE) program. CoDE provided abbreviated diabetes educational services at low-cost, which included one-to-one educational services with long-term follow-up integrated into the medical services of an existing community health clinic at the Central Dallas Ministries Community Health Services (CDM-CHS). One of the objectives was to improve the quality of diabetes care and health outcomes for clinic patterns established by the American Diabetes Association.

CDM-CHS was established in 1988 and included three full-time family practice physicians, one of which was fluent in Spanish, a class D pharmacy, and support personnel, medical assistants, and community health workers of which 70% were also bilingual. Those qualifying for the CoDE programs could have neither health insurance nor have any alternate source of health care. The program utilized a CoDE educator who helps the patient self-manage their disease and provides individual case management under direct physician supervision. The community health worker or *promotora* is bilingual, holds a high school equivalency certificate, and is certified by the State of Texas as a promotora. Certified diabetes educators and registered dieticians from RCDC trained the promotoras to work with the community. The program focused on several key steps to first identity the health disparities and to reduce the burden of diabetes in the underserved Hispanic population within this community.

During the first educational visit, the patient completed a demographic and medical history form, the Diabetes Quality of

Life Survey, and a diabetes knowledge test. Patients were provided a glucose monitoring device and testing strips, at no cost, and were trained in how and when to use the device. The second visit focused on developing a personal meal plan, which was individualized and appropriate to the language, culture, and educational level of the patient. At this point, the promotora identified eating patterns and helped to develop a daily caloric intake for the patient, not to lose weight, but to decrease the amount of excessive carbohydrates consumed from food and beverages. The third visit focused on prevention of both short-term and long-term diabetes complications the patient may face. Complications, such as blindness, kidney failure, nerve damage, heart disease, and limb amputation, which can result from poor diabetes control, were all discussed in detail with the patient. Also, patients were encouraged to engage in 150 minutes of physical activity each week. At the end of the third educational visit, the promotora and patient negotiated a single goal to improve their diabetes control and personal well-being. Quarterly assessments were set up, to allow the promotora the opportunity to discuss any results with the patient. During these assessments, meal plans and portion sizes were reviewed and revised, patients were encouraged to bring in food packages and labels so that, with the assistance of the promotora, they could learn how to properly quantify the product, for medical testing of their glucose levels and to discuss their medication compliance.

Those patients who were accepted into the program needed to ensure that they keep all scheduled appointments and were responsible to re-schedule any missed appointments. After three undocumented no-shows, patients were dropped from the study. Of those patients who were not in compliance, or those that attended for a period of at least 12 months, their baseline A1C was 8.22%. After six months, A1C level for this group dropped to 7.59%, and within 12 months dropped to 7.14%. However, of those patients who were in compliance, those who completed all of the CoDE educational visits had a beginning baseline A1C of 8.14%. After six months, the average A1C level dropped to 7.36%, and after 12 months, the average A1C was 7.00%. While these numbers appear to show promise, problems arose during the time frame allowed for this program. First, some of the participants dropped out of the program because of their lack of interest; second, some relocated to other cities or returned to their country of origin; third, some obtained health insurance and were no longer eligible to be in the CoDE program; and fourth, one patient resolved their secondary diabetes diagnosis. Although, CoDE was developed to be a culturally appropriate intervention, it needed to take into consideration the economic culture of the community, as well. For example, those that received alternative health insurance were dropped from the program were now left with no promotora to assist them in keeping up with meal plan, exercise programs, self-management of their disease, and quarterly glucose testing at the clinic. For those conducting the study in the CoDE failed to see that once you have obtained a person's trust, letting them go so easily, breaks a bond that may be hard to fix in the future.

An earlier study was conducted by researchers with the University of Texas at Austin, School of Nursing and The University of Texas Health Science Center at Houston, School of Public Health, in which they wanted to determine the effects of culturally competent intervention among Mexican-Americans with Type 2 Diabetes. It was found that four counties along the Texas-Mexico border are predominantly populated by Mexican-Americans also have the highest diabetes-death rates in Texas. The Starr County Border Health Initiative (1994-1998) primary emphasis was on providing intervention in accessible community-based sites and offering activities that reflected cultural characteristics and preferences of the participants. The researchers knew that this group had the most difficulty controlling their blood glucose levels for a variety of reasons. Many Mexican-Americans are underinsured or have no healthcare insurance and therefore must rely on family and *cuaranderos* (folk healers) for health advice and remedies; while others lack reliable transportation to health care facilities, maybe isolated from mainstream culture, and may experience language barriers to receive the care they need. Since traditional interventions have been ineffective among Mexican-Americans, the researchers wanted to look at more culturally competent approaches.

For the study, the researchers and Starr County employed bilingual Mexican-American nurses, dieticians, and community workers from the county, utilized videotapes of Starr County community leaders discussing their experiences with diabetes, and offered services in Spanish, which was the preferred language within this community. In conducting meetings with participants, they utilized community-based schools, churches, adult daycare centers, and community health clinics throughout the county. This helped to focus on the success for the participants, provided rapid and frequent feedback, promoted group problem-solving in addressing health questions and issues, and resulted in an increased network of support. Over a six-month and twelve-month period, lower levels of A1C and fasting blood glucose levels and higher diabetes knowledge scores were reported in the experimental group than those of the control group. Although the A1C levels for the experimental group were lower than the control group, the mean A1C levels were still considered higher than normal or above 7.0%. While the study showed mixed results, this study did confirm overall improved health outcomes when utilizing culturally competent approaches in health-related education and diabetes self-management among individuals within this Mexican-American community.

In Los Angeles, a similar grassroots program was initiated by Drs. Francine Kaufman and Anne Peters who wanted to combat the growing problem of obesity and Type 2 Diabetes. Working in separate clinics, but together in combating the problem, Drs. Kaufman and Peters joined forces in an effort "to prove you can improve the health of the poorest of the poor." Three days a week, Dr. Peters leads a team that cares for 2,000 working-class immigrant diabetics at a Los Angeles County-run clinic in predominately Latino East Los Angeles. Dr. Kaufman treats children, heads the Center for Diabetes, Endocrinology and Metabolism at Children's Hospital Los Angeles.

As a team, both doctors looked at why the disease ran higher in some communities, brainstormed to find possible solutions that could be tailored to these communities, and in the process identified several key issues that provide roadblocks in addressing the health needs within these communities.

Both doctors identified one of the problems within these communities was they had few grocery stores, with fresh fruits and vegetables and an oversupply of fast-food restaurants, which sell low-cost, high-fat, high-carbohydrate, and high-calorie products. They found that it was far easier to tell your patient to eat healthy, and much more difficult for that patient to find places to buy healthy foods to consume. Drs. Kaufman and Peters also identified, what they believed were, cultural barriers that lead to higher rates of obesity within this community. First, fast food was identified as a status symbol, especially among new immigrant groups of all races. The ability to buy fast food showed that you had enough disposable income to provide this type of food for your family. Second, the fear of food shortages, led to many eating more food than they needed at each meal. Many believed that because the food was available now, it might not be available tomorrow, they needed to stock up. This was validated by many of their patients stating that there were times within the previous year they had to go hungry at least once because of economic hardships. Lastly, many parents did not see their children as having a weight problem. Many parents in the community believed their children did not have a problem with their weight, although nearly two-thirds of them qualified as being overweight or obese. Parents of babies they called "their little butterball" insisted that their child was healthy and were actually concerned that the child was not eating enough.

In 1997, Congress established the Special Diabetes Program for Indians, which was developed to address the growing diabetes epidemic among American Indians and Alaska Natives. The Indian Health Service (IHS), Division of Diabetes Treatment and Prevention provides $150 per year in grants for diabetes treatment and prevention services among the 399 IHS, Tribal, and urban

Indian health programs in all 12 IHS administrative areas across the US. Since 1998, 333 Community-Directed Diabetes Programs have been in place to provide diabetes treatment and prevention that address specific local priorities. As mandated by Congress, in 2004, 66 Demonstration Projects, which look at scientific findings and best practices from the research literature in real world settings and design and implement structured interventions to not only prevent diabetes, but to reduce the incidence and risk of cardio-vascular heart disease among Native Americans who are diagnosed with diabetes.

In the State of New Mexico, the Department of Health and Human Services—Indian Health Service (IHS) Division of Diabetes Treatment and Prevention administers the two grant programs. According to the IHS website, in 2006, New Mexico received approximately $7 million for 30 Community-Directed Diabetes Programs and approximately $2.5 million for 7 Demonstration Projects. In total, the State of New Mexico has received approximately $46.5 million for the Community-Directed Diabetes Programs and approximately $7.5 million for the Demonstration Projects. Many of the prevention and intervention programs utilize cultural appropriate techniques to help Native American children and adults understand how to self-manage their health problems. The community-directed program also ensures that IHS clinics can provide better services and treatment with the most up-to-date equipment. While these programs are showing some positive results in the education, treatment and prevention programs, diabetes among Native Americans continues to be a major issue.

In looking at culture and diet on the internet, I came across an Ohio State University Extension Fact Sheet produced by their Department of Family and Consumer Sciences. This fact sheet was entitled, Cultural Diversity: Eating in America, Mexican-American (HYG-5255-95), and was one in a series of nine developed to address the issues of cultural diversity in American eating patterns. The other eight in the series are African-American (HYG-5250-95), Amish (HYG-5251-95), Appalachian (HYG-5252-95), Asian (HYG-

5253-95), Hmong (HYG-5254-95), Middle Eastern (HYG-5256-95), Puerto Rican (HYG-5257-95), and Vietnamese (HYG-5258-95). What I found very interesting was the one statement in this paper, which also appears in each series.

"Cultural diversity is a major issue in American eating. To fully understand the impact cultures play in American nutrition, one must study both food and culture."

The Mexican-American fact sheet covers the traditional Mexican diet, which was impacted by economic and social factors such as income, education, urbanization, geographic regions, and family customs. This also looked into how the traditional Mexican diet changed with the large immigration of Mexican nationals to the United States. Healthy changes included increased consumptions of milk, vegetables, and fruits, with a decrease in lard and Mexican cream. However, with the introduction of salads and cooked vegetables, this increased the consumption of fats, with the addition of salad dressings, margarine, and butter. Another unhealthy diet change was the replacement of traditional fruit-based beverages with high-sugar processed drinks. Lastly, as Mexicans acculturated into American society, they began to eat less beans and rice and eat more highly processed inexpensive fast foods, which are higher in both fats and calories. So the traditional Mexican diet has been replaced by one that no longer resembles what their ancestors ate. This fact sheet goes into some detail about why it is important to understand culture, beliefs, norms, food practices, and terminology in order to better serve those that need assistance in managing their health education. It also goes into detail about the importance of family and family structure within the Mexican culture.

What I found, is that this fact sheet validated the cultural issues and the family traditions I felt would be needed when researching what the foods were of our peoples. These issues within our own combined cultural history became crucial when my husband and I created our individualized healthy eating plan. Ultimately, what these studies and examples tell me personally is no matter what approach you take, you need to be able to understand your culture, your family unit, including your friends, and your environment at home, and especially the commercial environment, including fast food restaurants and full service grocery stores.

One final thought about my journey in understanding food in the context of my culture, my family tradition, and the lifestyle changes in eating I needed to make. You need to keep your mind fresh, by reading articles about health research, food research, and even vitamin supplements. This will not only expand how you eat, but can give you a better understanding on the vast variety of foods that can become part of your tradition. Years earlier, I never thought that my being born and raised in Chicago, with my love of a variety of the ethnic foods of my hometown, that I would be so drawn to the foods of the southwest. It never occurred to me to look into the foods of my people as a resource to healthy eating and a satisfying lifestyle of choices in foods.

6

Recipes and Menu Options

Although my husband and I have, over the years of cooking, collected recipes that we prefer, we know that in some cases it is important to have a basic cookbook. So, it is important that you also have at least one or two cookbooks, on hand. This helps for a variety of reasons. First, this helps to expand your cooking base by providing numerous recipes that you may decide to include in your diet. Second, it gives you basic recipes so that you do not have to spend a lot of time thinking about how to prepare meals for your family. Third, the ingredients will be listed, so that you will know whether or not you would want to include this recipe and also whether you would take the opportunity to change the recipe to suit your own tastes. I have taken some of my favorite recipes from cookbooks, magazines, and other sources, such as family and friends.

Over the years, I have found that I have relied on several very basic cookbooks. My own personal preferences are the following: *Better Homes and Garden: Complete Step-by-Step Cookbook.* This was my very first cookbook I purchased because as a young wife and homemaker I felt I did not have enough cooking and baking experience in the kitchen. I purchased this particular cookbook in 1978 because it has the basics for almost every kind of cooking and baking technique. A few years ago, my sister-in-law sent me a handy little cookbook entitled, *So Fat, Low Fat, No Fat*, by Betty Rohde. This already has basic substitutions in the featured recipes and the recipes are already tested for success. My most recent find was a more personal cookbook entitled, *Foods of the Americas: Native Recipes and Traditions* by Fernando and Marlene Divina in association with the Smithsonian National Museum of the American Indian. This book helped my husband and me to rediscover more of the traditional foods of all Native American cultures. It contains many recipes that we knew about and recipes we had eaten in the past. It also contains recipes we had some general knowledge about, but unfortunately did not know how exactly to prepare. Because these cookbooks helped to expand our recipe base, we will always have new recipes to try.

I am always looking for cookbooks of interest because there is always room to expand your cooking base. Because of this, I found a book on the market that is almost identical to the Super Foods Rx (which features 14 Super Foods) and one I am considering adding to my personal collection. This cookbook entitled, *12 Best Foods Cookbook: Over 200 Delicious Recipes featuring the 12 Healthiest Foods*, by Dana Jacobi. This cookbook is interesting because of the 12 healthiest foods this cookbook features, 10 are part of the 14 super foods collection. Also, this book is interesting because it lists dark chocolate as a healthy food and provides recipes with this ingredient. Overall, I believe this cookbook may be a good companion book to the *Super Foods Rx*. One thing to remember, when following any recipe in any cookbook, not all recipes may be totally healthy. For example, meats that are high in saturated fats, the wrong fats and oils and highly processed sugars and grains may be required as part of the recipe. After reading the sections on food groups, you should know enough to be able to alter the recipes and make them healthier.

My husband and I have spent the past few years changing and updating the way we prepare some of our favorite traditional foods. These are just a few recipes to show you that with a little creativity you can prepare traditional foods in a healthier way. Some of these recipes are ones that we enjoyed as part of our combined tradition. Some were handed down from family members and some recipes we just made up because we enjoyed the different flavors and textures of the foods. My hope is that this will give you some ideas of your own and that you may even modify some of your family recipes better and healthier, and more to your own family's taste. Feel free to alter these recipes as you wish, keeping in mind the basic rules of healthy eating.

Main Dishes

Green Chili Stew (New Mexico style)

1 pound, fresh roasted and peeled long green chili (NOT JALAPENO)
or
1-16 oz. tub *Bueno* frozen green chili (hot or mild)
2 whole chicken breasts
1 small can fat free chicken broth
1 small can pinto beans (in place of potatoes)
2 tbsp. minced garlic
1-16 oz. bag shoepeg or supersweet white corn
1 tbsp. dry cilantro
1-16 oz. bag of sliced zucchini squash
salt to taste

Parboil chicken. Trim and discard fat (or give to your dog) and cut chicken into small cubes. While chicken is cooking, peel and clean out seeds from fresh green chili. Frozen green chili will already be peeled and de-seeded. In food processor on low speed, chop chili into medium to small pieces. Drain and rinse the pinto beans. In a non-aluminum stewing pot, place all the ingredients. (During the summer you may add fresh zucchini squash.) Add enough water to cover the ingredients. Bring to fast boil, then lower heat, cover and simmer for about 20-30 minutes.

Green Chili Enchiladas—Stacked (New Mexico style)

Green Chili Stew (see above recipe)
blue corn meal or cornstarch
1 whole chicken breast
corn tortillas
1-16 oz. pkg. Mexican style cheese (low-fat)

You can make the green chili stew or use the leftover stew from the day before. Boil the chicken breast in a separate saucepan. Trim and discard the fat (or give to your pet) and shred the chicken. Place in a non-aluminum medium saucepan and add some of the liquid from the stew and heat. In a non-aluminum Dutch oven, place the stew and heat. In a glass add 2-3 tablespoons of blue corn meal or cornstarch with 1-1 ½ cups of water and stir until mixed. Add this to the stew and heat to soft boil. Dip one tortilla into the stew for about 10-20 seconds to soften and warm. Remove and place flat on plate. Place shredded chicken on top and if you wish, sprinkle a little cheese (this will help keep the layers together). Heat a second tortilla in the stew and place on top of first layer. Completely cover stack with a heaping spoonful of stew. Sprinkle lightly with cheese. If you desire, you may place in microwave for about 25-30 seconds to completely melt the cheese.

Shrimp Gumbo

3-4 lbs cooked shrimp, tail off
8-10 strips pre-cooked bacon
½ cup uncooked wild rice
1 small can pinto beans or black beans
1 large can crushed tomatoes
1 tsp. *Tony Chachere's* Original Creole Seasoning
1-16 oz. bag supersweet white corn
1-2 cups chopped green chili
1 tbsp. olive oil (optional)
5 cups water

2 tbsp. minced garlic
1 tsp. *Old Bay* Seasoning
2 pkg. *Sazon Goya* with
    coriander and annatto
½ cup *Goya* Sofrito

1 bunch fresh cilantro,
    diced
½ onion, diced

Place uncooked wild rice in colander and rinse well in cold water (see rinsing method under wild rice section). Place in 6-quart slow cooker. Drain and rinse beans and add to slow cooker. Place all ingredients, except bacon, in slow cooker and stir well. Turn on high. Microwave pre-cooked bacon for about 30 seconds. Blot excess fat from bacon, chop and add to slow cooker. Cook on high for about 4-5 hours.

Or

Place uncooked wild rice in colander and rinse well in cold water. Place in medium stewing pot. Drain and rinse beans and add to pot. Place all ingredients, except bacon, in pot and stir well. Turn on medium high heat. Microwave pre-cooked bacon for about 30 seconds. Blot excess fat from bacon, chop and add to pot. Bring to boil, then lower heat and simmer for about 1 hour.

Laguna-Style Green Chili

1 pound of lean ground turkey	1 tbsp. olive oil
1-16 oz. bag supersweet white corn	2 tbsp. cilantro
1 large can red kidney beans	2 tbsp. minced garlic
1 large can stewed tomatoes	1 small onion, chopped
2 small cans tomato sauce	5 cups water
1 cup chopped green chili (hot or mild)	
1 pkg. Sazon Goya with coriander and annatto	
½ cup Goya Sofrito	

Brown turkey and drain any excess fat. Place in large Dutch oven. Drain and rinse kidney beans and add to turkey. Add remaining ingredients and turn on medium heat and bring to boil. Lower heat and simmer for about 30 minutes.

By simply adding a 16 oz bag of lima beans, 8 oz of dry whole-wheat macaroni noodles, and an extra cup of water you change the meal into a goulash.

Puerto Rican Chicken

3 lbs. chicken breast tenders
1 liter bottle of diet *Pepsi/Coke*/cola
1 large or 2 small cans of pinto beans
2 pkgs. *Sazon Goya* with coriander and annatto

1-16 oz. bag sliced carrots	1-6 oz. jar of *Goya* Sofrito
1-16 oz bag cut green beans	½ cup diced onions
1-14.5 oz. can crushed tomatoes	
in puree	1 tbsp. minced garlic
1 small can tomato paste	2 tbsp. canola oil

Parboil the chicken tenders, drain and rinse, trimming any excess fat. Set aside. In a stew pot, on medium heat, place the oil adding the onions and sauté until the onions are translucent. Add the garlic, tomato paste, tomato puree, Sofrito, Sazon seasoning, mixing well. Slowly add the diet cola (which ever brand you prefer), stirring constantly. Drain and rinse the beans and add to stew pot, along with the carrots, green beans, and parboiled chicken. Slowly bring to soft boil. Lower heat and simmer for about 30-45 minutes. Stir constantly, as mixture will slightly thicken as it cooks. Serve over steamed brown rice.

Pasticcio (Greek Lasagna)

Meat filling:

2 tbsp. *Smart Balance* Buttery Spread	2 tsp. salt
1 cup chopped onion	¼ tsp. pepper
2 lbs lean ground beef or ground turkey *	¼ tsp. cinnamon
1 small can tomato paste	½ cup fine dry
1 large or 2 small cans tomato puree	breadcrumb

Noodles:
1-16 oz. box of elbow macaroni
1-2 eggs or egg substitute equivalent

Egg Sauce topping:

1/3 cup *Smart Balance* Buttery Spread	¼ tsp. nutmeg
1/3 cup whole-wheat pastry flour	3 cups 1% or skim milk **
pinch of salt, pepper	
2 eggs or egg substitute equivalent	

To Prepare Meat filling:

In large pan melt butter and brown onions. Add ground meat, brown, and drain excess fat. Place on medium heat and add tomato paste, tomato puree, salt, pepper, and cinnamon and stir ingredients. Add breadcrumbs and mix thoroughly. Cover on low heat for 15 minutes until thickened.

To Prepare Noodles:

Cook macaroni and drain with cold water. Place in large bowl and when cooled, add eggs (substitute) and stir to cover noodles thoroughly. In a well-greased 9 x 12 glass lasagna pan, place half of the noodles and smooth out. Set the remaining noodles aside. Spoon ground meat mixture over the noodle layer, gently smoothing out. Place remaining noodles over the layer of meat and smooth out.

To Prepare Topping:

Over medium heat, melt butter, stir in flour, salt, pepper, and nutmeg. Slowly stir in milk a little at a time, each time blending milk into the mixture. Stir constantly, until sauce thickens and starts to boil. In a small dish slightly beat eggs. On low heat pour eggs (or substitute) into the sauce, stirring constantly until thickened and bring to a boil, but do not bring to a full boil. Quickly pour sauce over noodles. If you want, you may lightly sprinkle Parmesan cheese over the top. Bake at 350° for 45-60 minutes, uncovered. Let stand for at least 15 minutes before serving. Cut into squares and serve.

You can alter this recipe in several additional healthy ways:

In place of 2 lbs. meat, use 1 lb. ground beef or ground turkey and a small bag of spinach, chopped. After browning meat and draining any excess fat, add spinach and slowly cook, until it cooks down. Then add remaining ingredients.

In place of 1% or skim milk, you may use unsweetened plain soymilk. The soymilk will take longer to set, so the baking time will be closer to the 60 minutes.

Spicy Turkey Stew

8 oz. cooked turkey, diced	1 cup chopped green chili
1-16 oz. bag supersweet white corn	2 tbsp. cilantro
2 small cans pinto beans	2 tbsp. minced garlic
2 small cans tomato paste	4 cups water
1 small can tomato sauce	

Drain and rinse pinto beans and place in 4.5-quart slow cooker. Add remaining ingredients and place on high for about 3-4 hours.

Minestrone

1 small can black beans	½ cup onion, diced
1 small can tomato paste	1 tbsp. minced garlic
1 small can tomato sauce	1 tsp. Italian seasoning
2 cups mixed vegetables	1 tsp. olive oil
1 cup uncooked whole-wheat rotini	2-3 cups water
1 cup chopped celery	

Drain and rinse black beans and combine with remaining ingredients, except rotini, in slow cooker. Turn on high. In a saucepan, boil the rotini, then rinse and add to the slow cooker. Cook on high for about 2-4 hours.

Side Dishes

No Fuss Spicy Mexican Rice

1-10 oz. can *RoTel* Diced Tomatoes *   2 ½ cups water
2 cups brown rice   ½ tsp. ground cumin
1 pkg. *Sazon Goya* with cilantro and tomato

Place all the ingredients in a rice cooker and turn on. Most rice cookers have an automatic off button that stops cooking when rice is done (approximately 25-35 minutes).

*You may use *RoTel* Original, Extra Hot, Milder, Chunky, or Mexican Festival, or your preferred brand of diced tomatoes if you cannot tolerate hot/spicy foods.

You may also add 1 small can of sweet peas or diced mixed vegetables to add variety to the rice dish.

Pasta Salad

1-16 oz. box of whole-wheat rotini *
1 pkg. of turkey salami
1 each green, yellow, orange peppers
2-3 tbsp. McCormack's Salad Supreme
2 large tomatoes or 4 Roma tomatoes
1-16 oz. bottle Italian dressing
1 cucumber
1 small can sliced black olives

Boil rotini until fully cooked. Rinse pasta with cold water until water runs cold through pasta, and set aside in large bowl. Slice peppers and tomatoes into cubes, peel cucumber and slice in halves or quarter cubes, drain liquid from black olives, and slice turkey salami pieces in half. Add these to bowl with pasta and mix well. Sprinkle the Salad Supreme and ¾ bottle of dressing, mixing well. Place in refrigerator until ready to serve. The pasta may soak up some of the dressing, so before serving add the remaining bottle of dressing, mixing well.

You may use whatever type of pasta you like, such as elbow macaroni, shells, bowtie, even the tri-color pastas.

Whole Wheat Bread Stuffing

2-1 lb loaves *Nature's Own* 100% Whole Wheat Sugar Free Bread
1 lb. pkg. celery, diced
1 tsp. ground sage
1 medium onion, diced
1 tsp. ground oregano
1/3 cup *Smart Balance* Buttery Spread
½ tsp. ground bay leaves
1-1 ½ cups water
pinch of salt

Cube bread and place in single layers on cookie sheets. Toast in oven at 350° for approximately 15-20 minutes or until lightly browned. DO NOT BURN the cubes. Let cool and place in an extra large mixing bowl.

In frying pan, over medium heat, melt butter. Add diced celery and onions and sauté until onions are translucent. Add seasonings, mixing well. Add celery/onion mixture to bread cubes, mixing thoroughly. Add approximately 1 cup of water, mixing well. Grab a handful of stuffing and squeeze into a ball. Stuffing should hold shape. If it does not hold shape, add another ¼ - ½ cup water. This will easily stuff a 15-18 pound turkey.

Hint: I always use a turkey oven bag to roast my turkey. This prevents the constant need for basting, reduces the use of additional butter, and reduces the cooking time. The turkey and stuffing use the steam in the bag to retain the moisture.

Breads

Pizza Crust

2 ½ cups whole-wheat pastry flour ½ cup olive oil
1 ½ cups oat bran 1 ½ cups warm water *
½ tsp salt 1 pkg. rapid rising yeast

In measuring cup, place warm water and yeast, mixing well. Then set aside for about 5 minutes. (Water should be warm enough to activate the yeast, but not too hot, as this will de-activate the yeast and the dough will not rise.) In a large bowl combine the flour, oat bran, and salt. Add the olive oil to the dry ingredients and mix well. Add the water and yeast mixture. This dough should be slightly stickier than usual, as the oat bran will absorb the excess moisture as the dough rises. Allow the dough to rise for about 1 ½ - 2 hours. Roll out dough to desired thickness on floured surface, place on pizza cooking sheet, and place your favorite sauce and toppings.

Sweet Potato Tortillas

2 cups mashed sweet potatoes
1 ½ - 2 cups whole-wheat flour

This recipe uses leftover baked sweet potatoes that were turned into mashed sweet potatoes. The mashed potatoes were buttered to taste and texture (with approximately 1/8 cup of Smart Balance buttery spread), ½ cup of water and unseasoned (no salt, no pepper), so the ingredients listed above are approximations.

In a medium bowl with the sweet potatoes, add the whole-wheat flour until the dough reaches the proper texture. (It should be slightly stickier than regular flour tortilla dough.) Pinch off into 2-inch balls and set aside. With your fingers and using your palms, take each ball and slowly flatten (this will allow a novice tortilla roller to keep as round a tortilla as possible.) Roll out each on a floured surface. As you roll out, continue to lightly dust the dough with flour to prevent it from sticking to the rolling pin and surface. Place rolled out tortilla on heated flat griddle or pan for approximately 30-60 seconds each side. Serve warm. Makes approximately one dozen.

Wild Rice Corn Fritters

1 cup cooked wild rice
½ cup whole wheat flour
½ cup supersweet white corn
1/8 tsp. salt
¼ cup pine nuts (*pinons*)
1/8 tsp. garlic powder
¼ cup chopped green onions
1 tbsp baking powder
2 eggs or egg substitute equivalent
¼ cup chopped green chili*
¼ to ½ cup cold water
canola oil, for deep-frying
*optional

Mix rice, corn, nuts, onions, green chili, and egg in large mixing bowl and set aside. In a second bowl, mix all of the dry ingredients and add to the rice/corn mixture. Slowly add the water until you get the slightly sticky consistency you prefer. Heat oil in medium saucepan. Carefully place large heaping tablespoons of mixture into hot canola oil and deep-fry until golden brown, turning over once. Remove and place on paper towel to drain excess oil. Serve warm. Makes approximately 12 to 16 fritters.

Sweets

Pie Crust

2 cups whole-wheat pastry flour
1 level tsp. cinnamon
dash of salt

¾ cup shortening
½ cup cold water

Mix flour, salt, and cinnamon, slowly cut shortening into mixture until mixture resembles a coarse meal. Add water, a little at a time and knead lightly until dough is formed. Cut dough into two pieces, place in plastic wrap and refrigerate for about ½ hour. Remove and gently roll out dough. Makes 2–9" single pie crusts or 1–9" double pie crust.

Graham Cracker Pie Crust

1/3 pkg (7) *Mi-Del* 100% whole wheat graham crackers
1/3 cup Smart Balance buttery spread

In food processor, crumb the graham crackers and place in 9" pie tin. Melt buttery spread and mix with graham cracker crumbs until well moistened. Slowly and carefully spread on bottom and sides of pie tin and set aside.

Blueberry Pie Filling

1-16 oz. bag frozen blueberries*
2 tbsp. cornstarch
8 oz. pureed frozen sweet cherries
1 tbsp. stabilized rice bran
1 tsp. vanilla extract

Optional: You may add an artificial sweetener or evaporated cane juice, to taste.

In saucepan, over very low heat, defrost cherries. Place cherries in blender and puree. In saucepan, over very low heat, defrost blueberries, add pureed cherries, vanilla, cornstarch, and rice bran. Heat until thickened and place in pie shell. Cover with top crust, seal edges, and cut vents in top crust. Bake at 350° for approximately 40 minutes or until done.

*You can substitute blackberries for blueberries to make blackberry pie filling.

Quick Cherry/Walnut Pie Filling

2 cups 100% Concord grape juice   ½ cup chopped walnuts
1½ cups dried tart cherries
1-2 tbsp. cornstarch (to thicken)
Optional: 1 level tbsp. rice bran
¼ - ½ cup cold water

In mixing bowl, place the dried cherries in the Concord grape juice. Allow the cherries to reconstitute for about 30 minutes. Place in saucepan, over medium heat, and bring cherries to the point of boiling, and turn to low heat. Add the walnuts and rice bran, mixing well. In a small measuring cup, mix cornstarch with cold water, then add slowly to cherry mix, until desired thickness is achieved. Place in pie shell. Cover with top crust, seal edges, and cut vents in top crust. Bake at 350° for approximately 40 minutes or until done.

Oat Bran Shortbread

1 ½ cup oat bran   2 tbsp. vanilla
1/3 cup grapeseed oil   1 cup water
2 tsp. baking powder

Mix all ingredients in bowl. Place in a greased 9-inch cake pan. Bake at 350° for approximately 20 minutes or until done. Allow shortbread to cool, cut into small squares and serve with your favorite sliced fruit (blueberries, strawberries, peaches) and a small dollop of fat free or low fat whipped topping.

Greek Sno-Ball Cookies

1 lb. unsalted sweet butter*
¾ cup organic powdered sugar
8 ounces of chopped pecans
1/8 cup of *Metaxa* (Greek liqueur)
4 ½ cups whole wheat pastry flour or 2 lb box cake flour**

Remove butter from refrigerator and allow butter to soften. (You may also place butter in microwave for approximately 10-15 seconds to soften, but be careful not to melt.) Cream butter with Metaxa and add powdered sugar, mixing well. Add the flour one cup at a time, mixing, well. (**If you use cake flour from a box, you will use slightly less than the 2 lb. box. Add the flour a little at a time until you get the right consistency.) Then add the pecans. You should be able to roll pieces of the dough into 1-inch balls between the palms of your hands and the balls should hold the form. Place the balls on an ungreased cookie sheet. Bake at 350° for approximately 15-20 minutes. Allow cookies to completely cool before coating them with powdered sugar. If you do not allow the cookies to completely cool, the warm cookies will absorb the powdered sugar coating and they will not stay white. Makes approximately 10 dozen (120) cookies.

*You may use whatever type of unsweetened butter. For example, I substitute 1 lb. organic unsweetened butter spreads.

Although this recipe uses organic powdered sugar, which is made from organic evaporated cane juice and organic cornstarch, is not entirely within my rules. Because I only make this during the holidays, I always give away most of the batch in little personal cookie tins as gifts. However, I will set aside whatever is leftover (usually about a dozen) for my personal use as this cookie has always been a part of my family holiday tradition.

Miscellaneous

Spicy Onion Dip

4 cups yogurt, non-fat, plain
¼ cup dehydrated chopped onion
1 tsp. dried cilantro
½-1 tsp. *Tony Chachere's* Original Creole Seasoning
Dash of turmeric (optional)

In a bowl combine yogurt, onion, and cilantro. Slowly add Creole seasoning and mix well, to your desired taste. Place in refrigerator for at least ½ hour before serving to re-hydrate the onions. Try this dip with *Eatsmart* all natural snacks—*Snyder's of Hanover* Veggie Crisps or your favorite all natural or trans fat-free chips.

Spinach Dip

1 cup *Smart Balance* Light Mayonnaise *
1 cup fat free sour cream
1-8 oz. can water chestnuts, drained and chopped
1 pkg. dry vegetable soup mix
½ cup finely chopped green onions
1 16 oz. pkg. frozen chopped spinach

Defrost, drain and squeeze moisture from the spinach and place in a bowl. Combine remaining ingredients. Place in refrigerator and chill several hours before serving. Serve with raw vegetables, such as baby carrots, cauliflower, and/or broccoli, or serve in a round whole wheat bread bowl (made from a loaf of your favorite round bread). You can dress up the bowl by breaking up the inside the bread into pieces for dipping and placing these pieces around the bread bowl. *You can substitute *Smart Beat* nonfat mayonnaise dressing or your favorite dressing.

Basic Blueberry Smoothie

½ cup 100% orange juice
½ cup blueberries, fresh or frozen
1 cup plain nonfat yogurt, with live active cultures
½ cup cherries, fresh or frozen*

*You may add ½ cup of any other type of fruit and/or vegetable, but you may need to add more orange juice and yogurt to keep the texture smooth

If frozen fruits are used, slightly defrost before blending. Mix all the ingredients in a blender on medium speed, until smooth. Makes 2 servings. A lot of times you can make your own smoothie using whatever fruits or vegetables you prefer. The whole idea is to use different kinds in different combinations. This will ensure that you will expand your choices and give you a larger variety to choose from.

For example:

Strawberry/Banana Smoothie: ½ cup (fresh or frozen) strawberries, ½ to 1 banana, ½ cup orange juice, and 1 cup of plain nonfat yogurt.

Pumpkin Smoothie: 1 tablespoon 100% (canned) pumpkin, ½ cup low-fat milk, half a banana, and a dash of cinnamon (*Prevention*, October 2005).

Menu Options

Breakfast

My standard breakfast is a bowl of oatmeal or steel cut oats, with blueberries or sliced banana and walnuts. My husband and I usually "treat ourselves" to something different on the weekends or when traveling, but our breakfast is always similar to what is listed below.

Oatmeal or steel cut oats with (1 cup) blueberries and (1 oz) chopped walnuts or:

- ½ cup blueberries, half banana, walnuts
- ½ cup blueberries, ½ cup chopped strawberries, walnuts
- ½ cup blueberries with whatever other fruit or nuts you prefer

Whole-grain pancakes or whole-grain French toast with sugar-free syrup

- with pecans
- with blueberries or preferred fruit, such as strawberry, apple
- with small side (2) bacon OR sausage

Multi-grain oatmeal pancakes with sugar-free syrup

- with small side (2) bacon OR sausage

One egg or egg substitute, two slices of bacon OR two sausage links/patties, one slice whole grain toast

- with small fruit cup
- with sliced tomato and cottage cheese

Whichever breakfast you choose, your breakfast should always include:

One 6-8 oz. glass of 100% high pulp orange juice. This provides the necessary amounts of vitamin C and the high pulp variety provides additional healthy fiber.

1 ounce of walnuts or pecans provides both the healthy amounts of protein and fat your body requires. Also, this is one of the easiest ways to include nuts in your daily healthy eating plan.

Miscellaneous Notes

Both at home and away remember to adhere to portion control. You do not want to begin the day by over eating the recommended serving sizes within certain food groups and loading your system with unnecessary saturated fats and wrong carbohydrates.

At restaurants avoid the two, three, and four egg combo plates, the 8 oz. plus breakfast steak or pork steak offerings, multiple pork sides (2-4 bacon, 2-4 sausage) options, and fried hash brown potatoes. These foods create a protein and/or carbohydrate overload. Always choose the egg substitutes, whole grains (buckwheat pancakes, whole-wheat toast), fresh fruits (blueberries, strawberries), and healthy fats in nuts (walnuts, pecans) from the menu.

Lunch

I like to eat a simple and fast lunch that does not require a lot of preparation. I am quite content eating sandwiches of different sorts: peanut butter or peanut butter and jelly sandwich, low-fat organic turkey breast/chicken breast sandwich, or a tuna sandwich/salad. I always use 100% natural peanut butter with no added sugars, 100% natural jellies, jams, or preserves with no added sugars, lower-fat varieties of deli-style lunchmeats, spinach in place of lettuce, and 100% sugar-free whole-wheat bread. Also, I will eat leftovers from the previous evening dinner, such as soups, stews, pasta, and pizza.

A favorite local restaurant of mine serves a wonderful *caldo*, or Mexican-style beef soup. This soup has tender lean beef chunks, carrots, cabbage, zucchini, corn-on-the-cob, and is seasoned to perfection. This comes in two sizes, a small bowl and a large bowl, served with two small homemade corn tortillas. Although, I could easily eat the larger serving, I will always select the smaller size.

Another favorite restaurant serves chicken or beef fajitas, with fresh homemade corn tortillas, frijoles de olla (pinto beans cooked in a pot, not refried), rice, and guacamole. This particular restaurant has a salsa bar, which includes sliced lettuce, cucumbers, onions, limes, fresh chopped cilantro, and about eight types of salsa, from mild to extra hot, including whole jalapeno peppers. Another favorite restaurant serves vegetarian fajitas, which is just as satisfying as regular fajitas.

Whichever lunch you choose, your lunch should always include:

At least one to two 16 oz. glasses of water, with a lemon or lime wedge

Try to select the healthiest foods within the major food groups, such as fruits and vegetables in their natural state, whole grain bread, poultry and fish.

Miscellaneous notes:

Adhere to portion control. If you do not bring your lunch to work, this is the area that you can easily eat more than the recommended serving sizes within certain food groups. Not only are portion sizes pre-determined by the restaurant, you may often feel you need to eat everything on your plate.

If you have the choice of the full meal or a la carte, opt for the a la carte. With the meal, always choose the small side salad over the potato side. Ask to substitute extra vegetables in place of the rice side. Most restaurants will do this to please the customer.

Avoid the higher saturated fat, higher carbohydrate types of foods. For example, when eating at most Asian-style restaurants: eat less white rice, do not eat fried rice, and select the vegetables and stir-fried (not deep fried) chicken/shrimp entrees. At American-style restaurants: choose baked or broiled chicken and fish, do not eat beef or pork, select vegetables and salads as the sides, and whole grain or multi grain varieties of breads. Do not pick at the bread basket or chips and salsa. As tempting as they are, these can fill you up with empty calories.

Avoid fat-free salad dressing, as these can contain hidden additives that sabotage any healthy eating plan. Order the regular house (oil/vinegar-based), Italian-style salad dressings. The oils/fats will help your body absorb more of the healthy nutrients found in vegetables. Still, do not drown your salad with any salad dressing. Portion control is important.

When eating a higher calorie lunch, try to eat a lower calorie high fiber dinner. When I eat lunch at a restaurant, I am almost always too full for a regular dinner so I will usually opt for some variety of steamed vegetables. Never skip any meal. It is better to eat something light for dinner because you do not want to go to bed hungry or snack heavily before you retire.

Dinner

I am lucky because, most of the time, I have the luxury of spending part of the afternoon preparing for dinner. I will usually defrost something early in the afternoon. However, there are times when planning dinner is not always an easy decision. Some recipes included here (found in this chapter under Main Dishes), are a few of my personal favorites and ones that I will make often.

- ❖ Green chili stew (New Mexico-style)
- ❖ Green chili chicken enchiladas—stacked (New Mexico-style)
- ❖ Shrimp Gumbo
- ❖ Laguna-Style Green Chili
- ❖ Turkey or chicken Stew
- ❖ Pasticcio
- ❖ Baked chicken with lemon pepper seasoning or *Tony Chachere's* Original Creole Seasoning

- ❖ Baked Tilapia, salmon, or your favorite fish with lemon pepper seasoning or *Tony Chachere's* Original Creole Seasoning or with minced garlic and fresh rosemary
- ❖ Brown rice, brown Jasmine rice, or wild rice with sliced jicama, turnips, rutabagas or chopped kale in red or green curry. For a non-vegan dinner, add stir-fry sliced lean beef, pork, chicken, turkey, or shrimp

Whichever dinner you choose, your dinner should always include at least one to two 16 oz. glasses of water.

As in the recommendation with lunch, try to select the healthiest foods within the major food groups, such as fruits and vegetables in their natural state, whole grain breads, poultry and fish.

Once again, the key is portion control. You do not want to end the day by overeating and overloading your body with unnecessary calories. Preparing meals at home gives you the most control over what and how your meal is actually prepared and how much you consume.

Most people believe that they simply do not have the time to prepare a perfectly, healthy dinner that the entire family will enjoy. First, try to enjoy cooking and experimenting with your old recipes.

If your children are old enough, get them involved in dinner planning and preparation. For example, when visiting my sister-in-law and her family during the summer, and I choose to make a pizza, I will have my nieces help with the prep work for the toppings, such as cutting the green peppers, onions, opening and draining the can of black olives, mixing the sauce, and even rolling out the dough to make their own individual pizza. They also take orders and prepare pizzas for the rest of the family. Then you can slowly teach them how to help prepare other recipes.

I also use my crock pot/slow cookers for much of my cooking. Or I will bake in the oven. Simply add all the ingredients and let the meal cook itself. This is another easy area in which your children can help you prepare meals.

If eating dinner at a restaurant, follow the basic suggestions for lunch. Also important, do not eat too late in the evening.

Snacks

One of my favorite after dinner snacks is simply a sliced banana or a few sliced strawberries, with a few pieces of pecans or walnuts, a sprinkle of unsweetened shredded coconut and sugar-free dairy-free melted dark chocolate chips. I also enjoy a small bowl my own version of trail mix: *Kashi* Go Lean cereal with unsweetened coconut milk or as a dry trail mix, with a handful of roasted unsalted mixed nuts and dried cherries. On occasion, I will eat a whole grain cracker, such as *Sesmark* Sesame Thins and *Sesmark* Rice Crackers, *Blue Diamond* Nut Thins, or *Ak-Mak* 100% Whole Wheat Stone Ground Sesame Crackers, with a few slices of cheese. Eat any snack along with a nightly cup of any variety of your favorite tea, such as black, green, red (rooibos), white, or any herbal mixture.

When I have guests over, I will purchase *Barry's Bakery* French Twists, a sweet puffed pastry that is a non-dairy, no butter, no cholesterol, no egg, no yeast, low sodium, and trans fat free dessert. I have also found a variety of gluten-free and dairy-free desserts and snacks that are quite flavorful. Regardless of which type of dessert and snack you purchase, moderation and portion control are important when eating any of these products.

4 Hershey's sugar-free dark chocolate mini bars (approximately 1 oz. of chocolate).

2-4 sugar-free dark chocolate covered strawberries or sliced bananas.

2-4 Greek Sno-ball cookies (on special occasions only) with afternoon or evening coffee or tea.

Any type of fresh vegetables, such as carrot sticks, celery sticks, broccoli, and cauliflower with fat free sour cream or fat free dip OR a small bowl of grapes, any variety of fresh berries, sliced pineapple, melon or apple, orange, or pear slices.

Air-popped popcorn, sprayed very lightly with your favorite trans fat free, low calorie butter spray and lightly salted.

Whichever snacks you choose, your snacks should always include:

Whole fruits and vegetables, whole grain cereals, that are trans fat free and sugar free or low sugar, whole grain tortilla or potato chips or crackers, that are trans fat free.

Any dessert or snack should be a treat or reward for eating well during the day and not as an unconscious habit. This is where you can change your unhealthy "comfort" foods for healthier choices.

Portion control is extremely important in this area. You need to pay special attention because it is very easy to eat a whole bag of chips without even realizing it. As a recovering tortilla and potato chip addict, I know how easy this is to do. In the past, I have done this many times. Make sure you do not eat directly from the bag. Read the label to see exactly how many chips constitute a serving size and measure only the specific number. Place your portion in a small bowl and do not go back for seconds.

Avoid the higher saturated fat, higher calorie processed snack products. Although many of the potato and tortilla chips are trans fat free, they are however still high in calories because they are fried in oil.

The Journey Continues

A s I stated, I began my journey in the fall of 1999. I am still on my journey to health and healing. Partly because I am in a new city; with a new doctor and a new and hopefully improved lifestyle, I will continue to make progress. This new part of my journey feels right. This journey feels good.

I am still researching health and health-related issues and whenever I hear about a health study or report on the news, I am on the internet to read the full story. I also religiously check certain websites to keep informed about news on topics that apply to me and my family. I still get long distance calls from my sisters about things they want me to check on for them. Even though I feel that I am as informed as I will ever be, I am still interested in collecting articles on health and health-related issues.

Recently, I found an article that stated that fibromyalgia may not be a condition, but a real disease. A study of researchers in France stated they found that fibromyalgia may be linked to abnormalities of blood flow in the brain. Through the use of a brain imaging technique, called a SPECT (single proton emission computed tomography), the researchers found functional abnormalities in the brain, regarding cerebral blood flow, also known as brain perfusion. The greater the degree of brain perfusion was directly linked to the severity of symptoms reported by those suffering from fibromyalgia.

This brings this condition one step closer to being successfully managed and treated.

As for my blood levels, in January 2009 I was hopeful that they would be within the normal range, but I knew I would have problem since I had gained a few pounds. My fasting blood glucose was 90, which is excellent and means I am not a diabetic. My total cholesterol was 160, with my HDL or "good" cholesterol at 42, more excellent numbers and my low dose of Lipitor is helping me to control my cholesterol. However, my triglycerides were high at 421. In spite of this, my doctor did not place me on a fibrate, fenofibrate, or even a different class of statin. He did prescribe a new FDA approved natural drug, Lovaza, which is being recommended for those persons with very high triglycerides. Lovaza is an omega-3 acid ethyl ester, which contains active fatty acids that your body is unable to produce. These fatty acids, along with diet and exercise, are proven to lower very high triglycerides. Although, I am using a drug to help control my hyperlipidemia condition, I am glad that my new doctor has recommended a natural drug over the usual class of "statin" drugs.

Afterward, my husband and I had a serious talk about what we both did wrong during the past 6 months. While I have decided that I cannot be his "taster" of whole grain, sugar-free baked goods and pancakes, I still have to own my part of the blame. I tried to include the wrong kind of processed products into my diet, even though they fell within my rules. I need to be more vigilant about what I consume. One mistake I made was eating organic rice-based and soy-based, non-dairy vegan ice creams, which were lower in calories and carbohydrates. While I did not consume as much of these products as did my husband, I still found myself eating them several times a week. Although the sugar content was much lower than regular milk-based ice cream products and was a mixture of organic and natural sugars, they still contained sugar. In spite of this, I allowed these to quickly become a "comfort" food. I know I cannot do this and I knew they were not within my Second Rule of Eating — No to "OSE."

In my three month follow-up examination in April, my cholesterol, fasting blood glucose were both within the normal acceptable range, while my triglycerides dropped to 331. My doctor decided to keep me on Lovaza and Lipitor and continue to monitor my progress for another three months. Then in early June, my triglycerides dropped to 252 and all of my remaining blood levels were within normal and acceptable ranges. However, my doctor was still not happy with my "high" triglyceride levels. After discussing my options with me, he decided to make a few minor changes in my medication. He decreased my Lipitor to 10mg a day, but added 500mg of Gemfibrozil, a generic Lopid. Gemfibrozil was one medication that I had previously used in 2001, with little success. Although, we discussed my previous experience with the generic Lopid, my doctor felt taking Gemfibrozil, along with the Lipitor would prove to have more success. Then in October, all of my blood glucose levels still were within normal ranges, while my triglycerides dropped 47 points to 205. Although, my weight is higher than I would like, at 132—135 pounds, I have resolved myself to the fact that I will never be the "skinny" 90—105 pound teenager I was, or the thinner 115—120 pound woman of my 20s and 30s. So my new weight goal is to be at least below 130 pounds. At this point, my doctor is satisfied with my progress and continued to keep me on my current prescription medication plan, with another blood test ordered in the spring of 2010. From there, we will decide how to progress in my road to gaining complete control of my condition.

Although I am happier in my new city and my new home, I still had periods when I felt anxious and sad—so I ate. Also, I needed to come to the full realization that my husband can eat many foods that I cannot, because he does not have the same health problems I have. Just because I buy the product for him, does not mean I can be weak and eat these food products along with him. I am now resolved to put things in perspective and make the effort to follow my rules. I am still on the road to eating healthy, hiking with my dog every day, and trying to exercise on those days that I am not able to walk.

My husband's journey will always be a slightly smoother

journey than mine. His blood lipid levels have remained within the normal ranges and well within the acceptable ranges. Although, I am still on the road to being healthier, I know that I will always have to commit to make healthier decisions for myself. I will always hold the key to my health. Because of this, some things will remain the same. I will continue to be proactive in my health decisions and work along with my doctor to help in my journey to better health. I will continue my journey and walk the nutritional road of culture, health, and healing. I am still on my "I'm not on a diet" healthy eating plan and continue to take my natural supplements daily, along with vitamin supplements. And I will continue to exercise daily. This journey is not a temporary commitment. My journey is a lifelong commitment to a long and healthy life that I choose to enjoy.

Nikki's Story

Every summer my husband and I go camping on our 5-acre forest property in Benzie County in northern-lower Michigan. Over a two-month period, we stay on our property for several weeks at a time to get away from it all and to de-stress. Because our property has no electricity, we use a small propane stove to cook our meals. Whatever we eat has to be fast, easy and still maintain the integrity of our healthy diet and lifestyle choices. During our 2005 summer vacation, my husband's cousin, Vernon, and his wife, Claudia, were talking to us about how we were able to adapt our diet to a camp-style way of cooking meals. During the conversation, Claudia mentioned that her daughter, Nikki, who has Down syndrome, was having problems controlling her cholesterol, even with the cholesterol-lowering drugs prescribed by her doctor. Nikki is smart, independent, has the ability to work at a job she enjoys, and with a little help is able to budget her income. Because she lives in an assisted independent living community home, Claudia, her mother, was concerned that Nikki may not be eating enough healthy foods and did not know if Nikki would be willing to change certain eating habits.

After talking with them about our dual problems, the hidden additives that had negative effects on my past diets, and how we currently managed our diets, Claudia seemed to think that her daughter could benefit by making changes in her diet and by maybe trying to include some of my diet rules into her own lifestyle. Because the taste and texture of foods was important hurdle to overcome in Nikki's case, Claudia thought that some of my suggestions could prove to be difficult to include in Nikki's improved diet. Although in Claudia's favor, Nikki did like many foods that were part of my daily diet, such as whole wheat in breads and a large variety of fruits and vegetables. So after returning from vacation in mid-August, I sent Claudia a rough draft copy of Chapter Three, which contained my rules of eating and rules of shopping, along with a copy of the Super Foods Rx to use as a reference book. I felt that even if Claudia found it difficult to help Nikki accept and incorporate my rules that Claudia would at least benefit from reading the all the material I sent.

After reading my chapter and the book, Claudia began by replacing Nikki's "white" products by purchasing whole grains, such as whole wheat breads, oatmeal, and brown rice, and then began to eliminate the "ose" by purchasing sugar-free natural foods, such as natural peanut butter, fresh and frozen fruits and vegetables, and 100% fruit juices. Because she is incorporating my first and second "diet" rules—"white" is bad and no to "ose," she will naturally follow my first "shopping" rule—read the labels and my second and third "shopping" rules—generic is fine and frozen or canned is fine. Also, without realizing she is also starting to eliminate things with higher saturated fats and adding things that do not contain trans fats, which are my third and fourth "diet" rules—limit red meats and eat the right fats.

By including Nikki in this process of selecting newer products to use, Nikki became empowered and invested in her dietary decisions. After all, this is Nikki's healthier eating plan. Claudia told us that Nikki now tells her friends that they don't eat the "right" foods, because she easily recognizes what is not a healthier choice.

Claudia jokingly stated that Nikki has become a bit of a "food elitist" because she does not hesitate telling others that they don't eat healthy. Over the past several months, while continuing to take her medication, following her doctor's orders, and incorporating some of my rules to healthy eating, Nikki's cholesterol dropped approximately 50 points and she lost several pounds. Although Claudia felt a little discouraged that Nikki did not lose more weight, her doctor put these results in perspective. It is more important to focus on the fact that her cholesterol level was lowered and then more easily controlled, rather than focus on only losing weight. From the time of her winter 2005 doctor's visit to the summer of 2006, Nikki's cholesterol dropped an additional 15 points. She continues to stay on her journey to better health.

Some of the parents of Nikki's friends, that live with her in the assisted independent living community home, have asked Claudia what she did to get Nikki's cholesterol levels within a healthier range. She mentioned my rules and how she made some simple changes to Nikki's diet. I have told Claudia to feel free to share my rules with the other parents.

Seth's Story

Seth is a former student of Kip. I first met him during the "holiday buffet" the students held the last day of fall 2007 classes. During the buffet, I talked informally to a number of students about the food they brought and the food that I had made. I told them about why I prepared the dishes they way I did, touching lightly about my family history of Type 2 Diabetes. It was at this point that a few of the students mentioned similar problems within their own families. Seth mentioned his father's diabetes diagnosis, but had indicated that his father was a "controlled diabetic." I did not have the opportunity to go into a deeper discussion about his father.

In mid-March 2008, just before the spring break, Seth arrived at class looking a bit troubled, as if he had something on his mind, other than the class. Afterward, he told my husband that he had bad news.

He told Kip that his doctor told him his blood tests revealed he had extremely high cholesterol levels, slightly over 400. All of his other blood levels were normal. Because of his family history with Type 2 Diabetes, his doctor wanted to place him on cholesterol-lowering statins. He told Kip he had taken this news badly, and did not want to start taking prescription medication because he feared being on medication for the rest of his life—like his father. He felt that at age 41, he was going to lose the battle and eventually become an adult diabetic—like his father. Kip told Seth that he would bring him a copy of my book to read, in the hopes it would give him the starting point and the confidence he needed to gain control of this condition.

Two months later, at the end of the spring semester, Kip's students had to do a poster presentation in relation to a group project. Since I was invited, I had the opportunity to see how Seth was doing on his journey to finding good health. Although I did not consider Seth to be overweight, I was very happy to see a slimmer Seth. He had lost about 12 pounds and was working on a new goal of losing another 10. His cholesterol was well within the normal range. According to his doctor, who was very pleased with Seth's progress, he was no longer advising Seth to take the cholesterol-lowering medication. As we discussed his new goals, he mentioned that he was having trouble losing the last 10 pounds. I told him to not focus on his weight, to let his body tell him what weight it needed to be as long as his blood levels were normal, and that he had most likely hit the plateau everyone does in any weight loss program. I reminded him that he was now at a point where the weight would be lost more slowly and that if he lost any more weight it would take months, not weeks. He just needed to be patient with his goals. The last I heard, Seth is still working on his journey to healthy living and he now shares my book with other members of his family.

What I find most gratifying, is that through my own experience, I was able to help others overcome similar health-related problems. I believe that more people need to be aware that better dietary habits are not that difficult to incorporate into your lifestyle. I also want them to see that eating healthy is not a form of punishment, but can be an enjoyable and delicious alternative, especially when you include family and friends in a way which honors your culture and traditions. I believe that if you truly want to make the necessary changes in the way you eat, you need to come to your moment of "epiphany." This is when you realize that change is necessary and that you are prepared to make the change. I feel really good that I may have had the opportunity to make a positive impact on someone else's life.

References

Note: Websites were current at the time this book was published but may have changed.

Agatston, Arthur. *The South Beach Diet: The Delicious, Doctor-Designed, Foolproof Plan for Fast and Healthy Weight Loss*. New York: Rodale/St. Martin's Press, 2003.

Alley, Holly and Crawley, Connie. "Less Fat for the Health of It." University of Georgia, Cooperative Extension Service, 1997. www.healthgoods.com.

American Chemical Society (ACS). "Soda Warning? High-Fructose Corn Syrup Linked to Diabetes, New Study Suggests." *Science Daily*, 23 August 2003. www.sciencedaily.com.

American Diabetes Association (ADA). *Complications of Diabetes in the United States*. www.diabetes.org (accessed December 21, 2008).

American Diabetes Association (ADA). *Diabetes and Native Americans*. www.diabetes.org (accessed December 21, 2008).

American Diabetes Association (ADA). *Direct and Indirect Costs of Diabetes in the United States*. www.diabetes.org (accessed December 21, 2008).

American Diabetes Association (ADA). "Mexico Warns Diabetes May Bankrupt Health System." ADA: Reuters, *In Diabetes Today*, 3 August 2007. www.diabetes.org.

American Diabetes Association (ADA). *The Dangerous Toll of Diabetes*. www.diabetes.org (accessed December 21, 2008).

American Diabetes Association (ADA). *Total Prevalence of Diabetes and Pre-Diabetes*. www.diabetes.org (accessed December 21, 2008).

American Diabetes Association (ADA). *Type 2 Diabetes Complications.* www.diabetes.org (accessed December 21, 2008).

American Dietetic Association (ADA). *Shop Smart—Get the Facts on Food Labels.* The American Dietetic Association Knowledge Center, Nutrition Fact Sheets, 2009. www.eatright.org (accessed May 20, 2009).

American Heart Association (AHA). *Fatty Fish Cuts Risk of Death from Heart Attack in Elderly.* 1 March 2001. www.americanheart.org.

American Heart Association (AHA). *Heart Disease and Stroke Statistics.* 2008 Update. www.americanheart.org.

American Heart Association (AHA). *Heart Facts 2007: Latino/Hispanic Americans.* 2007 Update. www.americanheart.org.

American Heart Association (AHA). *Reading Food Labels.* Updated 10 December 2007. www.americanheart.org (accessed January 10, 2008).

American Institute for Cancer Research (AICR). *Foods That Fight Cancer.* Updated 2005. www.aicr.org.

American Obesity Association (AOA). *Obesity—A Global Epidemic.* AOA Fact Sheets, Updated 2 May 2005. obesity1.tempdomainname.com (accessed May 20, 2009).

American Obesity Association (AOA). *Obesity in Minority Populations.* AOA Fact Sheets, Updated 2 May 2005. obesity1.tempdomainname.com (accessed January 4, 2009).

American Obesity Association (AOA). *Obesity in the U.S.* AOA Fact Sheets, Updated 2 May 2005. obesity1.tempdomainname.com (accessed May 20, 2009).

Anderson, James W., Elizabeth C. Konz, and David J.A. Jenkins. "Health Advantages and Disadvantages of Weight-Reducing Diets: A Computer Analysis and Critical Review." *Journal of the American College of Nutrition*, Vol. 19, No. 5 (2000): 578-590.

Archuleta, Martha. "Fitting Meat, Poultry, and Fish into a Healthy Diet, Guide E-129." New Mexico State University (NMSU), College of Agriculture and Home Economics, Cooperative Extension Service, January 2003.

Atkins, Robert C. *Dr. Atkins' New Diet Revolution.* New York: Avon Books (Mass Market PB)/HarperCollins, 2002.

Australian Nut Industry (ANI). *Nuts For Health*, Horticulture Australia Limited, ANI Fact Sheets, 2003: www.nutsforhealth.com.au.

A1C Handout: [LAN-PD-4256-1 (072)]. Bridgewater, NJ: Aventis Pharmaceuticals, Inc., 2002.

Balch, Phyllis A. *Prescription for Nutritional Healing: A Practical A-Z Reference to Drug-Free Remedies Using Vitamins, Minerals, Herbs & Food Supplements*. 3rd edition. New York: Penguin Putnam, Inc., 2000.

Bantle, John P., S.K. Raatz, W. Thomas, and A. Georgopoulos. "Effects of Dietary Fructose on Plasma Lipids in Healthy Subjects." *American Journal of Clinical Nutrition*, November 2000, 72: pp. 1128-1134.

Batz Jr., Bob. "Hemp Milk? It's Healthy and Legal as Hemp Cereal." *Pittsburgh Post Gazette*, 2 May 2007. www.post-gazette.com.

Bellerson, Karen J. *The Shopper's Guide To Fat In Your Food: A Carry-Along Guide To The Fat, Calories & Fat Percentages in Brand Name Foods*. Garden City Park, NY: Avery Publishing Group, 1994.

Better Homes and Gardens. *Complete Step-by-Step Cook Book*. 1st edition, 7th printing. Des Moines, IA: Meredith Corporation, 1978.

Blumert, Michael and Jialiu Liu, MD. *Jiaogulan: China's "Immortality" Herb*. Third printing. Badger, CA: Torchlight Publishing, Inc., 2003.

Borushek, Allan. *The Doctor's Pocket Calorie, Fat, & Carbohydrate Counter*, 2004 Color Edition. Costa Mesa, CA: Family Health Publications, 2004.

Boyles, Salynn. "Obese, Diabetic Youths Have Artery Plaque." WebMD: Heart Disease Health Center, *WebMD Health News*, 26 May 2009. www.webmd.com.

Boyles, Salynn. "How Many People Will Have Cancer in 2030?" WebMD: Cancer Health Center, *WebMD Health News*, 30 April 2009. www.webmd.com.

Boyles, Salynn. "Fresh Take on Fructose vs. Glucose." WebMD: Metabolic Syndrome Health Center, *WebMD Health News*, 21 April 2009. www.webmd.com.

Boyles, Salynn. "High Fructose Corn Syrup's Bad Rap Unfair?" WebMD: Health & Cooking, *WebMD Health News*, 11 December 2008. www.webmd.com.

Boyles, Salynn. "Global Cancer Deaths to Double by 2030." WebMD: Cancer Health Center, *WebMD Health News*. 9 December 2008. www.webmd.com.

Brody, Jane E. "To Preserve Their Health and Heritage, Arizona Indians Reclaim Ancient Foods." San Pedro Mesquite Company, *The New York Times: Science Times*, 2001. www.spmesquite.com.

Brown, S.A., RN, PhD, FAAN, A.A. Garcia, RN, MSN, K. Kouzekanani, PhD, and C.L. Hanis, PhD. "Culturally Competent Diabetes Self-Management Education for Mexican-Americans: The Starr County Border Health Initiative." *Diabetes Care*, 25 (2002): 259-268.

Carroll, Jill. "The Government's Food Pyramid Correlates to Obesity, Critics Say." *The Wall Street Journal Online—Health*, 13 June 2002. www.karlloren.com.

Case, Verna. "Obesity: American Population Tips the Scales." North Carolina: Davidson College, Biology Department, Senior Colloquium, Biology 401, Fall 2008. bio.davidson.edu (accessed May 27, 2009).

Center for Disease Control (CDC). *Obesity Among Adults in the U.S.—No Statistically Significant Change Since 2003-2004.* CDC Data Brief Number 1, November 2007. www.cdc.gov (accessed November 28, 2007).

Center for Disease Control (CDC). *Trends in Diabetes Prevalence Among American Indian and Alaska Native Children, Adolescents, and Young Adults - 1990-1998.* CDC, National Center for Chronic Disease Prevention and Health Promotion, Publications and Products, Fact Sheet, Updated 20 December 2005. www/cdc.gov (accessed December 26, 2008).

Cicero, Karen. "15 Foods That Can Save Your Heart." WebMD: Heart Health Center, *WebMD Feature* from *Shape Magazine*. 1 February 2008. www.webmd.com.

Collins, Karen. *Nuts: A Health Food If Used Right.* American Institute of Cancer Research (AICR), 2001: www.diabeticgourmet.com.

Craig, Winston J., PhD, RD. "Phytochemicals: Guardians of Our Health." Berrien Springs, MI: Andrews University, A Continuing Education Article, 2005. vegetariannutrition.net (accessed November 18, 2008).

Culica, Dan, MD, PhD, James Walton, DO, and Elizabeth A. Prezio, MD. "CoDE: Community Diabetes Education for Uninsured Mexican Americans." Baylor University Medical Center, *Proceedings*, Vol. 20, Number 2 (2007), pp. 111-117.

Dairy Management, Inc. "Facts about Cheese." dairyinfo.com (accessed November 28, 2007).

DeMouy, Jane. *The Pima Indians: Genetic Research.* National Institute of Diabetes and Digestive Kidney Diseases (NIDDK). diabetes.niddk. nih.gov/dm/pubs/pima/genetic/genetic.htm.

De Noon, Daniel J. "Diabetes Slows Brain Function." WebMD: Diabetes Health Center, *WebMD Health News*, 5 January 2009. www.webmd. com.

De Noon, Daniel J. "U.S. Cancer Deaths, New Cancers Decline." WebMD: Cancer Health Center, *WebMD Health News*, 25 November 2008. www.webmd.com.

De Noon, Daniel J. "Diabetes Up 90% in U.S." WebMD: Diabetes Health Center, *WebMD Health News*, 30 October 2008. www.webmd.com.

De Noon, Daniel J. "Fatty Liver Disease: Genes Affect Risk." WebMD: Digestive Disorders Health Center, *WebMD Health News*, 26 September 2008. www.webmd.com.

De Noon, Daniel J. "Americans Fatter in 37 States." WebMD: Healthy Eating & Diet, *WebMD Health News*, 19 August 2008. www.webmd.com.

De Noon, Daniel J. "More Heart Deaths in Nation's Future?" WebMD: Heart Disease Health Center, *WebMD Health News*, 11 February 2008. www.webmd.com.

DiabetesSite.Net. "Diabetes among Native Americans." Updated 2005. www.diabetessite.net/native.html (accessed December 26, 2008).

DiabetesSite.Net. "Diabetes in Children and Adolescents." Updated 2005. www.diabetessite.net/children.html (accessed December 26, 2008).

DiabetesSite.Net. "How Many African Americans Have Diabetes?" Updated 2005. www.diabetessite.net/african.html (accessed December 26, 2008).

Dickerson, George W. "Nutritional Analysis of New Mexico Blue Corn and Dent Corn Kernels—Guide H-233."New Mexico State University (NMSU), College of Agriculture and Home Economics, Cooperative Extension Service, February 2003. www.cahe.nmsu.edu (accessed May 28, 2007).

Divina, Fernando and Marlene Divina. *Foods of the Americas: Native Recipes and Traditions*. In Association with the Smithsonian National Museum of the American Indian. Berkeley, CA: Ten Speed Press, 2004.

Edgar, Julie. "Western Diet is a Global Heart Risk." WebMD: Heart Disease Health Center, *WebMD Health News*, 20 October 2008. www.webmd.com.

Epic4Health. "Statins and Adverse Effects: CoQ10 and Statin Drugs." Updated 2003. www.epic4health.com/coqandstatdr.html (accessed June 23, 2005).

Epstein, Daniel. "Diabetes Higher on U.S.-Mexico Border." *Medical News Today*, 20 November 2004. www.medicalnewstoday.com.

Eskenazi, Rachel. "Fighting 'Inevitability' of Developing Type 2 Diabetes in Mexican-Americans." *Endocrine Today*. www.endocrinetoday.com (accessed December 30, 2008).

Favaro, Avis. "Simple Grain Offers Health Benefits to Diabetes." Canada: *CTVglobemedia*, 15 November 2007. www.ctv.ca.

Firshein, Richard N. *Reversing Asthma: Breathe Easier With This Revolutionary New Program*. New York: Warner Books, 1996.

Foreman, Judy. "Thyroid, Cholesterol Are Linked." *The Boston Globe: The Globe Online*, 14 March 2000. www.boston.com.

Fraser, Jessica. "Diabetes and Hispanic Americans: More than Just Genetics." Truth Publishing LLC, *NaturalNews.com*, 27 June 2005. www.naturalnews.com.

Gall, Stephanie. "An Updated Guide to Soy, Rice, Nut, and Other Non-Dairy Milks." Home & Garden Publications, *Vegetarian Journal*, January–March 2008. findarticles.com.

Gavin, Mary L., MD. "Deciphering Food Labels." *The Nemours Foundation, Kids Health*. Updated 2008. www.kidshealth.org.

George Mateljan Foundation. "The World's Healthiest Foods: How to Select the World's Healthiest Foods." Various dates 2001–2009. www.whfoods.com.

Gifford, Maria. "Get In The Game: How To Build Your Winning Diabetes Health Care Team." *Diabetes Forecast*, April 2008, pp. 51-53.

Gilbert, Sue and Fran Clinton. "Ten Reasons to Eat Dairy (And 20 Easy Low-Fat Ways to Do It)." *iVillage*, 22 July 1999. www.health.ivillage.com.

Gillette, Cynthia and Julie Garden-Robinson. "A Bushel of Reason to Eat Your Fruits and Vegetables." North Dakota State University, Extension Service, October 2000. www.ext.nodak.edu/food/bushel.htm.

Gorman, Christine. "How to Eat Smarter." *Time*, 20 October 2003, pp. 48-59.

Gorman, Christine. "Why So Many of Us Are Getting Diabetes." *Time*, 8 December 2003, pp. 59-67.

Govias, Gaynor D. *Sulfite Sensitivity*. American Academy of Allergy, Asthma, & Immunology: Allied Health: Articles of Interest, Updated 2005. www.AAAAI.org.

Grim, Charles W., DDS, MHSA. *Facts on Indian Health Disparities*. Indian Health Service (IHS)—Fact Sheet, January 2006.

Gupta, Sanjay, MD. "Dear (Food) Diary." *Time*, 4 August 2008, p. 70.

Gupta, Sanjay, MD. "Rethinking Organics." *Time*, 20 August 2007, p. 60.

Gupta, Sanjay, MD. "Spicing Up Your Life." *Time*, 3 May 2004, p. 92.

Hale, Ellen. "Junk Food Super-Sizing Europeans." *USA Today*, November 18, 2003, World Section (A), pp. 13A-14A.

Hansen, Lonnie and Melinda Hemmelgarn. "Enjoying the Harvest: Don't Let a Wild Game Meal Leave You Chewing The Fat." The Missouri Department of Conservation, Updated September 2004. mdc. mo.gov.

Hayes, Dayle. "Choosing a Rainbow of Produce" The Deaconess Billings Clinic, *Nutrition News*, 27 July 2001. www.billingsclinic.com.

Heller, Lorraine. "Kellogg Reveals Major Shift in Marketing Practices to Kids." Decision News Media SAS, *Foodnavigator-usa.com*, 14 June 2007. www.foodnavigator-usa.com.

Heller, Lorraine. "Kellogg to Face Lawsuit Over 'Junk Food' Ads to Kids." Decision News Media SAS, *NutraIngredients-usa.com*, 18 January 2006. www.nutraingredients-usa.com.

Hendrick, Bill. "Rates Coming Down for Heart Disease, Stroke Deaths." WebMD: Heart Disease Health Center, *WebMD Health News*, 15 December 2008. www.webmd.com.

Henkel, John. "Sugar Substitutes: Americans Opt for Sweetness and Life." *Food and Drug Administration (FDA) Consumer Magazine*, November–December 1999. fda.gov.

Hewitt, Ben. "Shaky Pyramid?" *American Way Magazine*, 1 June 2003. www.americanwaymag.com.

Hitti, Miranda. "Hot Tea May Raise Esophageal Cancer Risk." WebMD: Cancer Health Center, *WebMD Health News*, 26 March 2009. www. webmd.com.

Hitti, Miranda. "2007 World Cancer Deaths Top 7 Million." WebMD: Cancer Health Center, *WebMD Health News*, 17 December 2007. www.webmd.com.

How to Use Fruits and Vegetables to Help Manage Your Weight. Department of Health and Human Services, Center for Disease Control and Prevention [Brochure], 2005. www.cdc.gov (accessed November 28, 2007).

Iannelli, Vincent, MD. "Food Pyramid for Kids and Adults: Food Guide Pyramid Controversies." About.com Inc., Pediatrics, *The New York Times Company*, Updated 18 June 2008. pediatrics.about.com (accessed May 28, 2009).

International Wild Rice Association (IWRA). "Wild Rice History." 2005. www.wildrice.org/iwrawebsite/html/ or www.wildricehistory.html.

Islami, F., Pourshams, A., Nasrollahzadeh, D., Kamangar, F., Fahimi, S., Shakeri, R., Abedi-Ardekani, B., Merat, S., Vahedi, H., Semnani, S., Abnet, C., Brennan, C., Moller, H., Saidi, F., Dawsey,

S., Malekzadeh, R., and Boffetta, P. "Tea Drinking Habits and Esophageal Cancer in High Risk Area in Northern Iraq: Population Based Case-Control Study." *British Medical Journal*, 26 March 2002: 338, DOI.

Jacobi, Dana. *12 Best Foods Cookbook: Over 200 Delicious Recipes Featuring the 12 Healthiest Foods*. New York: Holtzbrinck Publishers, 2005.

Jaret, Peter. "Nutrition Labels: The Fast Track to Diet Health." WebMD: *WebMD Feature*, 30 October 2008. www.webmd.com.

Jaworski, Stephanie. "Basic Ingredients." *The JoyofBaking.com, A Baking Resource*, 2005. www.joyofbaking.com.

John Hopkins University–Medicine (JHUM). "Are Organic Foods Healthier?" 15 May 2008. health.yahoo.com/experts/nutrition.

John Hopkins University–Medicine (JHUM). "Fruits and Veggies: Fresh, Canned, or Frozen?" 11 April 2008. health.yahoo.com/experts/nutrition.

Jones, Kenneth. "The Potential Health Benefits of Purple Corn." *The Journal of the American Botanical Council, Herbal Gram*, 2005: 65: 46-49.

Kalinowski, Jennifer, MPH, RD. "Berry Good!" *Diabetic Living*, Summer 2005, pp. 80-89.

Kay, Leslie. "Phytochemicals at Work: Phytochemical Index," at the Nutrition Resource, LLC, Integrated Health Management, 1999. www.nutritionresource.com.

Kluger, Jeffrey. "How America's Children Packed on the Pounds." *Time*, 23 June 2008, pp. 66-69.

Ko Cruz, Mimi. "Fighting Obesity Across the Border." California State University, Fullerton, *Inside Magazine*, April 2008, p. 12.

Kohler, John. "The Truth about Agave Syrup: Not as Healthy as You May Think." *Living and Raw Foods*, 1998. www.living-foods.com.

Kovacs, Betty, MS, RD. "Fiber," *MedicineNet.com*, 2009. www.medicinenet.com.

Laino, Charlene. "Obese Kids Have Middle-Aged Arteries." WebMD: Heart Disease Health Center, *WebMD Health News*, 11 November 2008. www.webmd.com.

Lam, Michael, MD. "Pantothenic Acid and Pantethine." *LamMD.com, An Insider's Guide to Natural Medicine*, Updated 2002. www.drlam.com.

Leal Ferreira, Mariana and Gretchen Chesley Lang, eds. *Indigenous Peoples and Diabetes: Community Empowerment and Wellness*. Durham, NC: Carolina Academic Press, 2006.

Lee, Elizabeth. "Obesity Issue Spurs USDA to Revamp Food Pyramid."

Active Network, *The Atlanta Journal-Constitution*, 11 September 2003. www.active.com.

LePere, Renee. "It's The Kind of Carbohydrates, New Study Says." Sun Coast Media Group, Inc., *Sun and Weekly Herald*, 25 April 2004. pd/ sunherald.com.

Levenstein, Barbara. "How to Tell a "Good" Fat from a "Bad" Fat." *The Essential Fatty Acid (EFA) Quarterly Report*, Issue I:IV.

Levi, Jeff. "F as in Fat: How Obesity Policies are Failing America." *Trust for America's Health, Robert Wood Johnson Foundation*, August 2008.

Lewine, Howard, MD. "Another Culprit to Watch." *Newsweek*, 17 January 2005, p. 48.

Liebman, Bonnie. "The Whole Grain Guide" Center for Science in the Public Interest, *Nutrition Action Health Letter—US Edition*, March 1997. www.cspinet.org.

Longley, Robert. "Health and Human Service Awards Grant to Fight Obesity Among African Americans." Department of Health and Human Resources, *About.com—US Government Info*, April 2005. www.usgovinfo.about.com.

LoweringCholesterol.net. "Pantethine: Various Studies and Abstracts." Various dates. www.loweringcholesterol.net.

Magee, Elaine, MPH, RD. "Good Carbohydrates, Bad Carbohydrates: Why Carbohydrates Matter to You." WebMD: *WebMD Feature*, 20 October 2008. www.webmd.com.

Magee, Elaine, MPH, RD. "Keeping-It-Off Super Foods: 9 Foods That Can Help Keep the Extra Weight Away." WebMD: Health & Cooking, *WebMD Feature*, 24 July 2008. www.webmd.com.

Malkin, Elisabeth. "Mexico Confronts Sudden Surge in Obesity." *The New York Times*, 29 June 2005. www.nytimes.com.

Marchand, Lorraine H. *The Pima Indians: Obesity and Diabetes*. The National Institute of Diabetes and Digestive Kidney Diseases (NIDDK). diabetes.niddk.nih.gov (accessed December 21, 2008).

Mayo Clinic, Mayo Foundation for Medical Education and Research (MFMER). "Dairy Products: Selecting, Storing, and Serving." 2005. www.mayoclinic.com.

Mayo Clinic, Mayo Foundation for Medical Education and Research (MFMER)."Fibromyalgia." 25 June 2007. www.mayoclinic.com.

Mayo Clinic, Mayo Foundation for Medical Education and Research (MFMER). "Health Benefits of Chocolate?" 13 February 2004. www. mayoclinic.com.

Mayo Clinic, Mayo Foundation for Medical Education and Research (MFMER). "Reading Food Labels: Tips if You Have Diabetes." Updated 11 October 2008. www.mayoclinic.com (accessed January 13, 2009).

McGraw, Phil. *Dr. Phil's Ultimate Weight Solutions: The 7 Keys to Weight Loss Freedom*. New York: Free Press/Simon & Schuster, Inc., 2003.

Miraglio, Angela M., MS, RD. *Chocolate's Potential for Health Benefits*. Northbrook, IL: Weeks Publishing Company, May 2001. www.foodproductdesign.com.

Misner, Bill. "Killer Sugar! Suicide With A Spoon." *Pathway International*, 2001. www.immunebasics.com.

Murr, Andrew. "The Cultural War on Diabetes." *Newsweek*, 17 September 2007. msnbc.msn.com.

Nagel, Rami. "Agave Nectar, the High Fructose Health Food Fraud." Truth Publishing LLC, *NaturalNews.com*, 24 November 2008. www.naturalnews.com.

Nash, J. Madeline. "Obesity Goes Global." *Time*, 25 August 2003, pp. 53-54.

National Council of La Raza (NCLR). *Key Facts About Childhood Obesity in the Latino Community*. NCLR, Fact Sheet—2006. www.nclr.org.

New Mexico Department of Health (NMDH). *Diabetes and New Mexicans*. Updated 2006. www.health.state.nm.us.

New Mexico Department of Health (NMDH). *Diabetes in New Mexico: The Latest Facts—November 2007 Update*. NMDH, Diabetes Prevention and Control Program, Health Data Fact Sheet, November 2007. www.diabetesnm.org.

New Mexico Department of Health (NMDH). "The Prevalence of Health Conditions and Behaviors among Adults in New Mexico, 2006." NMDH, Diabetes Prevention and Control Program, Health Data. *New Mexico Epidemiology*, Volume 2008, Number 8. www.health.state.nm.us.

Nutrition and Health Services (NHS). *Nutrient Density Information*. US Department of Agriculture, Kentucky Department of Education, Division of NHS, Summer Food Service Program, 12 July 2005.

Ogilvie, Megan. "Oregano a Flu Fighter?" Toronto, Ontario, Canada: *Toronto Star Newspaper*, 30 January 2007. www.thestar.com.

On Line Media, S.A.E. "The 20 Super Foods." Updated 2003. cairodining.com (accessed December 1, 2008).

Park, Alice. "America's Health Checkup." *Time*, 1 December 2008, pp. 41-51.

Park, Alice. "Living Large." *Time*, 23 June 2008, pp. 90-92.

Park, Alice. "Stains "R" Us." *Time*, 21 July 2008, p.58.

Piccinin, Doris MS, RD. *More About Ethiopian Food: Teff*. Washington: University of Washington, Harborview Medical Center, Department of Nutrition and Food Service, April 2002. ethnomed.org.

Pick, Marcelle, OB/GYN NP. "Sugar Substitutes and the Potential Danger of Splenda." *Women to Women*, Updated 19 December 2008. www.womentowomen.com.

Plutkowski, Shelley. "The Skinny On Cooking Oils." *Mayo Clinic, Mayo Foundation for Medical Education and Research*, 27 July 2001. www.mayoclinic.com.

Pollard, Janet M., MPH, Mary K. Bielamowicz, PhD, RD, LD, CFCS, and Carol A. Rice, PhD, RN, eds. Various articles related to sugar substitutes. Texas A&M System, Texas AgriLife Extension Service, *Health Hints*, April 2006, vol. 10, No. 3, pp. 1-9.

Pratt, Steven and Kathy Matthews. *Super Foods Rx: Fourteen Foods That Will Change Your Life*. New York: HarperCollins Publishers, Inc., 2004.

Produce for a Better Health Foundation (PBH). "Why 5 A Day The Color Way." Updated 2005. www.5aday.com/.

Railey, Karen. *Whole Grains: Teff (Eragrostis)*. Earl, NC: Health and Beyond Online, 2008. www.chetday.com.

Rhoads, Caroline S., MD. "Diabetic Retinopathy—Topic Overview." WebMD: Diabetes Health Center, Medical Reference from *Healthwise*, Updated 13 April 2007. diabetes.webmd.com.

Rohde, Betty. *So Fat, Low Fat, No Fat*. 1st Fireside Edition. New York: Simon & Schuster, Inc., 1995.

Schafer, Elisabeth, Diane Nelson, and Christa Burton. "The Health Value of Fruits and Vegetables—PM 1855." Iowa State University of Science and Technology, Cooperative Extension Service, July 2000. www.extension.iastate.edu.

Simopoulous, Artemis P. and Jo Robinson. *The Omega Diet: The Lifesaving Nutritional Program Based on the Diet of the Island of Crete*. New York: HarperCollins, 1999.

Sonberg, Lynn. *The Quick & Easy Fat Gram & Calorie Counter*. New York: Avon Books, 1992.

Sorgen, Carol. "5 Super Foods for Your Heart: Every Heart-Healthy Diet Should Include These Foods." WebMD: Healthy Eating & Diet, *WebMD Feature*, 28 August 2008. www.webmd.com.

Spalter-Roth, Roberta, Teri Ann Lowenthal, and Mercedes Rubio. "Race, Ethnicity, and the Health of Americans." Sidney S. Spivack Program in Applied Research and Social Policy, *American Sociological Association*, Summary—July 2005.

Squires, Sally. "Sweet But Not So Innocent? High-Fructose Corn Syrup May Act More Like Fat Than Sugar With the Body." *The Washington Post, Nutrition and Health Section*, 11 March 2003, p. HE01.

Strange, Carolyn J. "Eat Smart for a Healthy Brain." WebMD: Healthy Eating & Diet, *WebMD Feature*, 18 December 2008. www.webmd.com.

Swancutt, Judy. "Is Your Cholesterol Too High? What Type of Fat Do You Eat?" *Health Care Partners*, 11 November 2001. www.experienceseniorpower.com.

Trowbridge Filippone, Peggy. "What is Butter Milk? Does Butter Milk Contain Butter?" About.com, Inc., The New York Times Company, *About.com: Home Cooking*, 2009. homecooking.about.com.

Trust for America's Health, Robert Wood Johnson Foundation. "New 2009 Report: Adult Obesity Rates Rise in 37 States, Obesity Rates Now Exceed 25 Percent in More Than Half of States." August 2008. www.rwjf.org (accessed January 4, 2009).

Underwood, Anne and Jerry Adler. "Diet and Genes." *Newsweek*, 17 January 2005, pp. 40-48.

United States Department of Agriculture (USDA). *The Food Pyramid Guide*. USDA, Home & Garden Bulletin Number 252, 1996. www.usda.gov.

United States Department of Agriculture (USDA). *Food Safety of Farm Raised Game*. USDA, Food Safety and Inspection Service Fact Sheets, April 2004. www.fsis.isda.gov.

United States Department of Agriculture (USDA). *Inside the Pyramid*. Updated 2005. www.mypyramid.gov.

United States Department of Agriculture (USDA). *MyPyramid Food Guidance System*. Updated 2005. www.mypyramid.gov/global_nav/media_questions_print.html.

United State Department of Health and Human Services (US DHHS). *Overview of Diabetes in Children and Adolescents*. US DHHS, National Diabetes Education Program (NDEP) Fact Sheet, August 2008. www.yourdiabetesinfo.org.

United States Department of Health and Human Services (US DHHS). *Diabetes and African Americans*. US DHHS, The Office of Minority Health (OMH), 27 June 2008. www.omhrc.gov.

United States Department of Health and Human Services (US DHHS). *Diabetes and American Indians/Alaska Natives*. US DHHS, The Office of Minority Health (OMH), 27 June 2008. www.omhrc.gov.

United States Department of Health and Human Services (US DHHS). *Diabetes and Hispanic Americans*. US DHHS, The Office of Minority Health (OMH), 27 June 2008. www.omhrc.gov.

United States Department of Health and Human Services (US DHHS). *Special Diabetes Program for Indians: New Mexico*. US DHHS, Indian Health Service (IHS), Division of Diabetes Treatment and Prevention, June 2008. www.omhrc.gov.

United States Food and Drug Administration (US FDA). *US FDA/CFSAN — How to Understand and Use the Nutrition Facts Label*. US FDA: Center for Food Safety and Applied Nutrition (CFSAN), November 2004. www.cfsan.fda.gov.

University of Michigan Health System (UMHS). "Spice Up Your Health in 2007 With These Savory Tips." *UMHS Press Release*, 2 January 2007.

University of Michigan Integrative Medicine (UMIM). "UMIM: Healing Foods Pyramid." University of Michigan Integrative Medicine Clinical Services, 2005. www.med.umich.edu/umim.

Wallis, Claudia. "Guess What F is For? Fat." *Time*, 15 September 2003, pp. 68-69.

Walsh, Bryan. "It's Not Just Genetics." *Time*, 23 June 2008, pp. 70-80.

Warner, Jennifer. "Diabetes Rates Rise in Older Population." WebMD: Diabetes Health Center, *WebMD Health News*, 28 January 2008. www.webmd.com.

Warrix, Marissa. "Cultural Diversity: Eating in America, Mexican-American," [Fact Sheet HYG-5255-95]. *Ohio State University Extension*, Family and Consumer Sciences, 1995. ohioline.osu.edu.

WholeHealthMD. Various articles. Sterling, VA: WholeHealthMD.com, LLC., *Reference Library: Foods*, (2004–2008). www.wholehealthmd.com.

Wilbert, Caroline. "Fibromyalgia a 'Real' Disease, Study Shows." WebMD: Fibromyalgia Health Center, *WebMD Health News*, 3 November 2008. www.webmd.com.

Wisegeek.com. "What Is Coconut Milk?" wisegeek.com (accessed January 17, 2010).

Wysong, R.L., MD. "Rationale for Nutritious Fats and Oils." Midland, MI: Wysong Corporation, 2005, pp. 1-7. www.wysong.net.

Zelma, Kathleen M., MPH. "10 Everyday Super Foods." WebMD: Healthy Eating & Diet, *WebMD Weight Loss Clinic-Feature*, 4 December 2008. www.webmd.com.

Lightning Source UK Ltd.
Milton Keynes UK
UKHW010645130621
385409UK00001B/73